Study Guide for

Basic Pharmacology for Nurses

Seventeenth Edition

Michelle J. Willihnganz, MS, RN
RCTC Nursing Instructor
Rochester Community and Technical College
Rochester, Minnesota

ELSEVIER

ELSEVIER

3251 Riverport Lane
St. Louis, Missouri 63043

Study Guide for Basic Pharmacology for Nurses, Seventeenth Edition   978-0-323-39611-0

Library of Congress Cataloging-in-Publication Data

Content Strategist: Nancy O'Brien
Content Development Manager: Jean Sims Fornango
Content Development Specialist: Laura Selkirk
Publishing Services Manager: Julie Eddy
Senior Project Manager: Mary Stueck
Design Direction: Renée Duenow
Publishing Services: Lisa Hernandez

Printed in the United States of America

Last digit is the print number: 9 8 7 6 5 4 3 2 1

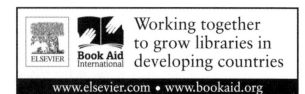

To the Student

This study guide was created to assist you in achieving the objectives of each chapter in *Basic Pharmacology for Nurses, Seventeenth Edition*, and establishing a solid base of knowledge in nursing pharmacology. This study guide has been completely revised to emphasize the chapter objectives with NCLEX-style questions. Completing the questions for each chapter in this guide will help to reinforce the material studied in the textbook and learned in class. Such reinforcement also helps students to be successful on the NCLEX-PN.

STUDY HINTS FOR ALL STUDENTS

Ask Questions!

There are no stupid questions. If you do not know something or are not sure, you need to find out. Other people may be wondering the same thing but may be too shy to ask. The answer could mean life or death to your patient. That is certainly more important than feeling embarrassed about asking a question.

Chapter Objectives

At the beginning of each chapter in the textbook are objectives that you should have mastered when you finish studying that chapter. Write these objectives in your notebook, leaving a blank space after each. Fill in the answers as you find them while reading the chapter. Review to make sure your answers are correct and complete. Use these answers when you study for tests. This should also be done for separate course objectives that your instructor has listed in your class syllabus.

Key Terms

At the beginning of each chapter in the textbook are key terms that you will encounter as you read the chapter. The key terms are in color the first time they appear significantly in the chapter. Phonetic pronunciations are provided for terms that students might find difficult to pronounce. The goal is to help the student reader with limited proficiency in English to develop a greater command of the pronunciation of scientific and nonscientific English terminology. It is hoped that a more general competency in the understanding and use of medical and scientific language may result.

Key Points

Use the Key Points at the end of each chapter in the textbook to help with review for exams.

Reading Hints

When reading each chapter in the textbook, look at the subject headings to learn what each section is about. Read first for the general meaning. Then reread parts you did not understand. It may help to read those parts aloud. Carefully read the information given in each table and study each figure and its caption.

Concepts

While studying, put difficult concepts into your own words to see if you understand them. Check this understanding with another student or the instructor. Write these in your notebook.

Class Notes

When taking lecture notes in class, leave a large margin on the left side of each notebook page and write only on right-hand pages, leaving all left-hand pages blank. Look over your lecture notes soon after each class, while your memory is fresh. Fill in missing words, complete sentences and ideas, and underline key phrases, definitions, and concepts. At the top of each page, write the topic of that page. In the left margin, write the key word for that part of your notes. On the opposite left-hand page, write a summary or outline that combines material from both the textbook and the lecture. These can be your study notes for review.

Study Groups

Form a study group with some other students so you can help one another. Practice speaking and reading aloud. Ask questions about material you are not sure about. Work together to find answers.

References for Improving Study Skills

Good study skills are essential for achieving your goals in nursing. Time management, efficient use of study time, and a consistent approach to studying are all beneficial. There are various study methods for reading a textbook and for taking class notes. Some methods that have proven helpful can be found in *Saunders Student Nurse Planner: A Guide to Success in Nursing School*. This book contains helpful information on test taking and preparing for clinical experiences. It includes an example of a "time map" for planning study time and a blank form that the student can use to formulate a personal time map.

ADDITIONAL STUDY HINTS FOR ENGLISH AS SECOND-LANGUAGE (ESL) STUDENTS

Vocabulary

If you find a nontechnical word you do not know (e.g., *drowsy*), try to guess its meaning from the sentence (e.g., *With electrolyte imbalance, the patient may feel fatigued and drowsy*). If you are not sure of the meaning, or if it seems particularly important, look it up in the dictionary.

Vocabulary Notebook

Keep a small alphabetized notebook or address book in your pocket or purse. Write down new nontechnical words you read or hear along with their meanings and pronunciations. Write each word under its initial letter so you can find it easily, as in a dictionary. For words you do not know or for words that have a different meaning in nursing, write down how they are used and sound. Look up their meanings in a dictionary or ask your instructor or first-language buddy. Then write the different meanings or usages that you have found in your book, including the nursing meaning. Continue to add new words as you discover them. For example:

primary
- of most importance; main: *the primary problem or disease*
- the first one; elementary: *primary school*

secondary
- of less importance; resulting from another problem or disease: *a secondary symptom*
- the second one: *secondary school (in the United States, high school)*

First Language Buddy

ESL students should find a first-language buddy – another student who is a native speaker of English and who is willing to answer questions about word meanings, pronunciations, and culture. Maybe your buddy would like to learn about your language and culture also. This could help in his or her nursing experience as well.

Contents

Drug Definitions, Standards, and Information Sources

chapter
1

Answer Key: Textbook page references are provided as a guide for answering these questions. A complete answer key is provided to your instructor.

MATCHING
Match the drug schedule on the right with the drug name on the left.

Drug

1. _____ diazepam (Valium)
2. _____ guaifenesin (Robitussin AC)
3. _____ heroin
4. _____ hydrocodone and Tylenol (Norco)
5. _____ methylphenidate (Ritalin)

Drug Schedule (U.S. Only)

a. Schedule I
b. Schedule II
c. Schedule III
d. Schedule IV
e. Schedule V

REVIEW QUESTIONS

Differentiate among the chemical, generic, and brand names of drugs.

6. The chemical names of drugs are used to: *(2)*
   1. describe the exact chemical makeup of the drug.
   2. provide a simpler way to identify the drug being manufactured.
   3. market the drug to the public.
   4. identify illegal drugs.
7. The generic names of drugs are used to: *(1)*
   1. describe the exact chemical makeup of the drug.
   2. provide a simpler way to identify the drug being manufactured.
   3. market the drug to the public.
   4. identify illegal drugs.
8. The brand names of drugs are used to: *(2)*
   1. describe the exact chemical makeup of the drug.
   2. provide a simpler way to identify the drug being manufactured.
   3. market the drug to the public.
   4. identify illegal drugs.

Identify the various methods used to classify drugs.

9. While studying drugs in school, the nursing student learns that the methods used to classify drugs includes their: *(Select all that apply.)* *(2)*
   1. chemical action.
   2. effect on a body system.
   3. therapeutic use.
   4. clinical indication.
   5. route of administration.

10. Examples of drugs that are classified by their physiologic or chemical action include: *(Select all that apply.)* *(2)*
    1. anticholinergics.
    2. antacids.
    3. antibiotics.
    4. beta-adrenergic blockers.
    5. antihypertensives.
11. When drugs are classified according to body systems, their effect can involve the: *(Select all that apply.)* *(2)*
    1. cardiovascular system.
    2. respiratory system.
    3. nervous system.
    4. apothecary system.
    5. metric system.

Identify sources of drug information available for healthcare providers.

12. Which resources are the most useful for nurses seeking information about prescription medications? *(Select all that apply.)* *(3)*
    1. Natural Medicines Comprehensive Database
    2. *Physician's Drug Reference*
    3. American Hospital Formulary Service, Drug Information
    4. Drug Interaction Facts
    5. Drug Facts and Comparisons
13. Which would be considered a reliable database for drug information that a nurse can consult? *(Select all that apply.)* *(4)*

1. *Handbook of Nonprescription Drugs: An Interactive Approach to Self-Care*
2. *United States Pharmacopeia (USP)/National Formulary (NF)*
3. Lexi-Comp
4. Electronic databases such as CINAHL
5. ePocrates

14. A patient has been experiencing adverse effects from a hypertensive medication he was prescribed. The nurse realizes that a reliable source to review prescription drugs and to report adverse effects in the MedWatch program is: *(3)*
    1. the *American Drug Index*.
    2. the *United States Pharmacopeia/National Formulary*.
    3. pharmacology textbooks.
    4. the *Physician's Drug Reference*.

15. A nurse is preparing a scholarly publication on the responses to and adverse effects of heparin. The most efficient and effective means of gathering information for this publication is to use: *(4)*
    1. package inserts.
    2. a consumer health website.
    3. Wikipedia.
    4. CINAHL database.

16. As a healthcare professional, it is important that the nurse determine the most accurate and up-to-date Internet information available for drugs, such as: *(Select all that apply.)* *(4)*
    1. ePocrates.
    2. DailyMed.
    3. Yahoo.
    4. Lexi-Comp.
    5. Krames Online.

Cite sources of credible drug information on the Internet.

17. A patient asked the nurse where to find information about the drug she was prescribed. The best response would be: *(4)*
    1. "Ask your healthcare provider to discuss your case in detail. The Internet can be misleading."
    2. "The best source for drug information is to just Google it."
    3. "We will give you all of the information you will need about your medications; you do not have to look any further."
    4. "A variety of sources are available to you. We will provide information, you can ask your physician, and you can research information online."

18. Credible sources of drug information on the Internet include: *(4)*
    1. Health on the Net Foundation.
    2. Micromedex.
    3. Wikipedia.
    4. DailyMed.

19. The nurse was explaining to a patient the various sources for drug information on the Internet site DailyMed, which has a searchable database that allows users to get more information when searching by: *(Select all that apply.)* *(4)*
    1. product name.
    2. indications for the drug.
    3. warnings.
    4. changes to the drug.
    5. active and inactive ingredients.

Discuss the difference between prescription and nonprescription drugs.

20. While studying the difference between prescription and nonprescription drugs, the nursing student needs to remember that prescription drugs: *(2)*
    1. are generally cheaper than nonprescription drugs.
    2. need to be obtained through a licensed healthcare provider.
    3. are identified using the brand name and nonprescription drugs use the generic name.
    4. do not have any serious side effects.

21. A patient asks the nurse what the difference is between prescription and nonprescription drugs. What is the best response by the nurse? *(2)*
    1. "The difference between the two classifications is really complicated and you just need to follow your doctor's advice."
    2. "Any store that has medications on the shelves indicates that you can purchase them without any doctor's order or prescription."
    3. "The difference between these two types of drugs is that one is the brand name and the other is the generic name."
    4. "Nonprescription drugs do not need to be approved by the FDA and prescription drugs do."

22. Healthcare providers who are licensed to prescribe drugs include: *(Select all that apply.)* *(2)*
    1. pharmacists.
    2. nurses.
    3. physicians.
    4. dentists.
    5. physician's assistants.

Describe the process of developing and bringing new drugs to market.

23. Those patients who participate in "testing in humans" are part of which phase of new drug development? *(6)*
    1. Preclinical research and development stage
    2. Clinical research and development stage
    3. New drug application review
    4. Postmarketing surveillance

24. The phase of drug development dealing with the therapeutic value and whether the drug appears to be safe in animals is known as: *(6)*

1. preclinical research and development stage.
2. clinical research and development stage.
3. new drug application review.
4. postmarketing surveillance.

25. The Black Box warning indicates that a drug that has already gotten FDA approval may have an: *(8)*
    1. associated risk of causing serious or life-threatening adverse effects.
    2. extremely high cost associated with it.
    3. effect that may cause nausea and vomiting.
    4. equally effective alternative drug.

Differentiate between the Canadian *chemical* name and the *proper* name of a drug.

26. The nurse is discussing the names of drugs with a patient in Canada, explaining that the difference between the chemical drug name and the proper name is the: *(9)*
    1. chemical name identifies the manufacturer.
    2. proper name of the drug is also the generic name of the drug.
    3. proper name is most meaningful to the patient.
    4. chemical name identifies the drug as recreational.

27. The *proper name* of a Canadian drug refers to the: *(9)*
    1. generic name of the drug.
    2. manufacturer.
    3. classification of the drug.
    4. chemical property of the drug.

28. A nurse was explaining to a patient that the difference between the generic name of the drug and the proper name is that: *(9)*
    1. the official name will be difficult to pronounce.
    2. generally there is no difference between the two names.
    3. the proper name is easy to remember.
    4. the proper name is usually the generic name of the drug.

Basic Principles of Drug Action and Drug Interactions

chapter

2

Answer Key: Textbook page references are provided as a guide for answering these questions. A complete answer key is provided to your instructor.

MATCHING

Match the route of administration on the right with the medication on the left. Routes will be used more than once.

Medications

1. _____ oral acetaminophen (Tylenol)

2. _____ subcutaneous insulin (Aspart)

3. _____ intravenous furosemide (Lasix)

4. _____ albuterol (Ventolin) nebulizer

5. _____ sublingual ondansetron (Zofran)

Route of Administration

a. percutaneous

b. enteral

c. parenteral

REVIEW QUESTIONS

Identify common drug administration routes.

6. The nurse knows that drugs are administered by which three most common routes? *(Select all that apply.)* **(14)**
   1. Enteral
   2. Distribution
   3. Percutaneous
   4. Parenteral
   5. Liberation

7. The enteral route includes medications administered: **(14)**
   1. subcutaneously.
   2. orally.
   3. transdermally.
   4. intravenously.

8. The nurse is explaining to the patient that the drug insulin given as a subcutaneous injection is best absorbed: **(14)**
   1. after the patient has eaten a meal.
   2. when deposited into the correct tissue.
   3. if the peripheral circulation is impaired.
   4. when a lump remains at the site of injection.

Identify the meaning and significance of the term *half-life* when used in relation to drug therapy.

9. A measure of the time required for elimination of a drug from the body is the: **(15)**
   1. expiration time.
   2. half-life.
   3. circulation time.
   4. minimum life.

10. The nurse knows that the drug alprazolam (Xanax) has a half-life of 12 hours, which means that how much drug will be left circulating in the body after 24 hours? **(16)**
    1. 50%
    2. 25%
    3. 30%
    4. 15%

11. The half-life of a drug may become considerably longer in patients who have: *(Select all that apply.)* **(16)**
    1. impaired kidney function.
    2. decreased thyroid function.
    3. impaired immune system.
    4. impaired liver function.
    5. decreased amounts of hemoglobin.

Describe the process of how a drug is metabolized in the body.

12. List in order the five stages that all drugs go through after they have been administered. **(14)**
    1. _____ Metabolism
    2. _____ Distribution
    3. _____ Excretion
    4. _____ Liberation
    5. _____ Absorption

13. How fast drugs are transferred from the site of entry into the body to the circulation is dependent on which factors? *(Select all that apply.)* **(15)**

1. Adequate amounts of fluid (usually water) when given orally
2. Deposited into the correct tissue when given parenterally
3. A lump remains at the injection site when given subcutaneously
4. Reconstituted with the correct diluent recommended by the manufacturer
5. How fine the droplet particles are for inhaled drugs

14. Drugs are rapidly dispersed throughout the body when administered by which route? *(14)*
    1. Oral
    2. Subcutaneous
    3. Intravenous
    4. Topical

Compare and contrast the following terms that are used in relationship to medications: *desired action, common adverse effects, serious adverse effects, allergic reactions,* and *idiosyncratic reactions.*

15. What is a *desired* drug action? *(17)*
    1. The predictable/usual response to the drug
    2. An unusual or idiosyncratic response to a drug
    3. A response capable of inducing cell mutations
    4. The unpredictable/unusual response to the drug

16. The nurse notices that the patient frequently complains about feeling queasy after taking her morning medications. This response could be termed a(n): *(17)*
    1. desired effect.
    2. serious adverse effect.
    3. common adverse effect.
    4. idiosyncratic reaction.

17. Patients who have allergic reactions from an administered drug typically experience which signs/symptoms? *(Select all that apply.)* *(18)*
    1. Severe itching
    2. Hives
    3. Diarrhea
    4. Respiratory distress
    5. Abdominal pain

Identify what is meant by a drug interaction.

18. Drug interactions are said to occur when: *(Select all that apply.)* *(18)*
    1. one drug enhances the pharmacologic effect of another drug.
    2. one drug inhibits the absorption of another.
    3. drugs are administered together.
    4. the action of one drug is altered by the action of another drug.
    5. drugs cause living cells to mutate.

19. A drug is considered pharmacologically active when it is: *(18)*
    1. bound to plasma proteins.
    2. unbound to plasma proteins.

3. distributed evenly throughout the body.
4. metabolized by the liver.

20. What resources can the nurse use to aid in determining when a drug interaction will occur? *(Select all that apply.)* *(19)*
    1. Consult with the pharmacist.
    2. Look up possible reactions in drug reference books.
    3. Ask the patient when he or she expects the drugs to interact.
    4. Memorize all possible drug interactions.
    5. Administer each drug several hours apart to ensure nothing happens.

Differentiate among the terms: *additive effect, synergistic effect, antagonistic effect, displacement, interference,* and *incompatibility.*

21. When a combination of two drugs will provide a greater effect than the sum of the effect of each drug if given alone, it is called a(n): *(19)*
    1. additive effect.
    2. antagonistic effect.
    3. synergistic effect.
    4. displacement.

22. The effect of one drug interfering with the effect of another drug is called: *(19)*
    1. additive effect.
    2. synergistic effect.
    3. antagonistic effect.
    4. displacement.

23. A common drug interaction that inhibits the metabolism or excretion of a second drug, thereby causing increased activity of the second drug, is called: *(19)*
    1. interference.
    2. incompatibility.
    3. antagonistic effect.
    4. additive effect.

24. When two drugs that have similar action are taken for an increased effect, this is termed: *(19)*
    1. antagonistic effect.
    2. displacement.
    3. synergistic effect.
    4. additive effect.

25. The drugs ampicillin and gentamicin are said to be incompatible because: *(19)*
    1. ampicillin displaces gentamicin from protein-binding sites.
    2. ampicillin inactivates gentamicin.
    3. ampicillin inhibits the excretion of gentamicin.
    4. ampicillin induces enzymes to metabolize gentamicin.

26. The term *displacement* refers to the drug-drug interaction that causes the first drug to: *(19)*
    1. inhibit the metabolism of the second drug.
    2. become unbound by the second drug, which increases the effect of the first drug.
    3. increase the effect of the second drug.
    4. decrease the half-life of the second drug.

Identify one way in which alternatives in metabolism create drug interactions.

27. What occurs as a result of enzymes becoming inhibited from metabolizing a drug? *(18)*
    1. Drug interactions
    2. Incompatibility issues
    3. An increase in protein-bound drugs
    4. Decreased absorption rates
28. When the metabolism of a drug is inhibited, then serum drug levels increase and may lead to: *(19)*
    1. displacement.
    2. bound drugs.
    3. toxicity.
    4. incompatibility.
29. When administering an enzyme inducer, the rapidly metabolized drug should be: *(19)*
    1. generally decreased.
    2. generally increased.
    3. remain at the same dose.
    4. discontinued.

Drug Action Across the Life Span

chapter

3

Answer Key: Textbook page references are provided as a guide for answering these questions. A complete answer key is provided to your instructor.

MATCHING

Match the correct definition of a drug action with the key term.

	Key Term		Definition of a Drug Action
1.	_____ placebo	a.	the use of multiple drugs for chronic illness that increases risk of drug interactions
2.	_____ tolerance	b.	drugs that cause birth defects
3.	_____ polypharmacy	c.	what drugs are attached to that are circulated in the blood
4.	_____ protein binding	d.	a drug form that has no active ingredients
5.	_____ teratogens	e.	when a person needs a higher dose to produce the same effect

REVIEW QUESTIONS

Explain the impact of the placebo effect and nocebo effect.

6. The nurse is explaining to a patient who is entering into a research study that he may actually get a placebo. Which statement by the patient indicates an understanding of the placebo effect? *(22)*
   1. "I will get the drug that they are testing for my condition."
   2. "I could possibly get a pill that will have a negative effect on my condition."
   3. "The placebo is a drug that has no active ingredients."
   4. "The placebo will have the same effect as the real drug."

7. The difference between the placebo effect and the nocebo effect is the: *(Select all that apply.) (22)*
   1. nocebo effect has occurred because the patient had negative expectations about the therapy.
   2. placebo effect has occurred because the patient had negative expectations about the therapy.
   3. nocebo effect has occurred because the patient had positive expectations about the therapy.
   4. placebo effect has occurred because the patient had positive expectations about the therapy.
   5. nocebo effect has occurred because the patient had no particular expectations about the therapy.

8. The attitudes and expectations of the patient regarding the treatment of his or her condition play a ma-

jor role in a patient's response to therapy. The nurse understands this to mean that patients with: *(22)*
   1. chronic silent conditions such as hypertension are more likely to adhere to the therapy prescribed.
   2. conditions such as arthritis are least likely to adhere to the therapy prescribed.
   3. conditions that have rapid consequences if therapy is not followed are more likely to adhere to the therapy prescribed.
   4. previous negative experiences are more likely to adhere to the therapy prescribed.

Identify the importance of drug dependence and drug accumulation.

9. Drug dependence occurs when the patient is: *(23)*
   1. unable to ingest drugs.
   2. indicating adequate pain relief from opioids.
   3. considered incompetent to make any medical decisions.
   4. develops withdrawal symptoms if the drug is discontinued.

10. The nurse suspects the patient has become dependent on the drug oxycodone because the patient: *(23)*
    1. asks for pain medicine more frequently than ordered.
    2. is groggy and hard to arouse about an hour after his dose.
    3. indicates adequate pain relief with the dose.
    4. is worried about becoming addicted to oxycodone and therefore will not take it.

11. When a patient becomes groggy and hard to arouse after receiving a dose of morphine, the patient may be experiencing drug: *(23)*
    1. dependence.
    2. tolerance.
    3. accumulation.
    4. withdrawal.

Discuss the effects of age on drug absorption, distribution, metabolism, and excretion.

12. In relation to drugs and the aging process, the nurse knows which is true? *(23)*
    1. Drugs have the same rate of absorption, distribution, metabolism, and excretion as people age.
    2. Drugs will have the same rate of absorption as people age, but their excretion will be affected by changes in the kidneys.
    3. The liver will increase its ability to metabolize drugs as people age.
    4. Pathologic conditions may alter the rate of drug absorption, distribution, metabolism, and excretion.

13. The nurse who takes care of children must remember that: *(23)*
    1. oral tablets are the easiest dose form to administer.
    2. subcutaneous injections will be the most dangerous drug route to administer.
    3. transdermal drug doses are the most difficult route of administration.
    4. liquid medications are the easiest dose form to administer.

14. Crushing medications for ease of administration in the elderly is often done, and is considered safe when giving: *(23)*
    1. enteric-coated tablets.
    2. sublingual tablets.
    3. tablet and capsule forms.
    4. timed-release tablets.

Explain the gender-specific considerations of drug absorption, distribution, metabolism, and excretion.

15. Drug absorption is influenced by the difference in men and women's: *(Select all that apply.)* *(24)*
    1. gastric motility.
    2. gastric emptying time.
    3. enzyme activity.
    4. saliva production.
    5. gastric pH.

16. Drug distribution is influenced by the difference in men and women's: *(Select all that apply.)* *(24)*
    1. amount and quantity of fat tissue.
    2. protein binding.
    3. gastric emptying time.
    4. cardiac output.
    5. regional blood flow to the target organ.

17. Drug metabolism is influenced by the difference in men and women's: *(Select all that apply.)* *(25)*
    1. hereditary characteristics or genes.
    2. number of active receptor sites.
    3. age.
    4. general health.
    5. maturity of the enzyme systems.

18. Drug excretion is influenced by the difference in men and women's: *(Select all that apply.)* *(25-26)*
    1. renal tubule function.
    2. evaporation through the skin.
    3. exhalation from the lungs.
    4. fat distribution in the body.
    5. GI tract motility.

List the definitions of the older use-in-pregnancy categories A, B, C, D, and X.

19. When a drug is listed as category C for use in pregnancy, this means: *(30-31)*
    1. the drug is safe to give during pregnancy.
    2. there have been no adequate studies done on the drug for use during pregnancy.
    3. the drug has a demonstrated risk to the fetus noted in studies.
    4. the drug is contraindicated for use during pregnancy.

20. A pregnant mother asks the nurse what is meant by "category A" for use in pregnancy. The nurse's response is: *(31)*
    1. "That means the drug is safe to take while you are pregnant."
    2. "Category A means that there have been no adequate studies done on the drug to determine if the drug is safe to take while pregnant."
    3. "That means the drug is contraindicated while pregnant."
    4. "Category A means that the drug has demonstrated a risk to the fetus during studies."

21. While reviewing medications prior to administration, the nurse notes that one drug was listed under category X for use in pregnancy, and remembered that this meant: *(31)*
    1. the drug had no supporting evidence to be used during pregnancy.
    2. the drug was safe to give during pregnancy.
    3. the drug was contraindicated during pregnancy.
    4. the drug was determined to have risks associated with fetal development.

Describe where a nurse will find new information about use of drugs during pregnancy and lactation.

22. A new nurse was talking with a seasoned nurse about changes in drug labeling. The seasoned nurse mentioned that the pregnancy categories have changed and to look up the new information in these websites: *(Select all that apply.)* *(31)*
    1. e-Pocrates
    2. Lexi-Comp

3. LactMed
4. HealthNet
5. DART

23. Databases such as TOXNET were developed for healthcare providers to: *(31)*
    1. gather information on drugs associated with increased risk to nursing infants.
    2. refer patients for more information regarding safe medications during pregnancy.
    3. review animal studies that are conducted on medications to determine safety issues.
    4. serve as a database for journals covering teratology and reproductive toxicology.

24. Which website is a resource for healthcare providers regarding information on drugs during pregnancy and lactation? *(31)*
    1. DailyMed
    2. NANDA
    3. DART
    4. MedMD

Discuss the impact of pregnancy and breastfeeding on drug absorption, distribution, metabolism, and excretion.

25. The nurse knows that a nursing mother has been taking paroxetine (Paxil) and has explained to her that taking this drug: *(32)*
    1. will interfere with the metabolism of a nursing infant.
    2. has an unknown effect, but may be of concern for a nursing infant.
    3. is associated with significant effects on nursing infants.
    4. is reported to have adverse effects on nursing infants.

26. It is safe to take medications during pregnancy and while breastfeeding if the drug is: *(32)*

1. labeled by the FDA as safe.
2. an herbal product.
3. known to be teratogenic.
4. nonprescription only.

27. A general principle that can be applied to pregnant women with regard to drug therapy is: *(32)*
    1. all drugs are safe during pregnancy.
    2. no drugs are safe during pregnancy.
    3. only drugs that have been approved by the FDA are safe during pregnancy.
    4. all herbal products have been determined as safe during pregnancy.

Discuss the role of genetics and its influence on drug action.

28. *Genetics* refers to the study of how living organisms inherit the characteristics or traits of their ancestors such as: *(Select all that apply.)* *(32)*
    1. hair color.
    2. body build.
    3. food preferences.
    4. enzyme systems.
    5. drug compatibilities.

29. Drugs are affected in the body by how enzyme systems: *(33)*
    1. metabolize them.
    2. excrete them.
    3. distribute them.
    4. absorb them.

30. Genetic polymorphisms are the naturally occurring variations in the structures of genes and are important in pharmacology because they: *(33)*
    1. cause more drug interactions or drug toxicity.
    2. will impact drug metabolism and excretion.
    3. will become teratogenic.
    4. create side effects from drugs.

The Nursing Process and Pharmacology

chapter

4

Answer Key: Textbook page references are provided as a guide for answering these questions. A complete answer key is provided to your instructor.

MATCHING

Match the type of nursing action on the right with the example of nursing action on the left. Types will be used more than once.

Example of Nursing Action

1. _____ reviewing a medication order
2. _____ determining when to turn a patient in bed
3. _____ obtaining the patient's medication history
4. _____ collaborating with the prescriber when to give a medication
5. _____ formulating an appropriate nursing diagnosis
6. _____ determining the frequency of drug administration

Type of Nursing Action

a. independent nursing action
b. interdependent nursing action
c. dependent nursing action

REVIEW QUESTIONS

Discuss the components and purpose of the nursing process.

7. Nurses use the nursing process to: *(35)*
   1. provide a framework for consistent nursing actions.
   2. assign nursing staff to patients.
   3. standardize the language nurses use to analyze nursing care.
   4. solve problems in nursing systematically.
8. An important aspect of the framework of the nursing process is that it uses: *(35)*
   1. an intuitive approach.
   2. a problem-solving approach.
   3. a scientific approach.
   4. an analytical approach.
9. List in order the steps used in the nursing process: *(36)*
   1. _____ Nursing diagnosis
   2. _____ Evaluation
   3. _____ Assessment
   4. _____ Planning
   5. _____ Implementation
10. The nurse considers the patient's psychosocial and cultural needs during which step of the nursing process? *(36)*
    1. Assessment
    2. Planning
    3. Nursing diagnosis
    4. Implementation

11. The nurse uses which step of the nursing process to detect any potential complications? *(36)*
    1. Assessment
    2. Planning
    3. Nursing diagnosis
    4. Implementation

Explain what the nurse does to collect patient information during an assessment.

12. Nurses perform the task of patient assessment to determine: *(Select all that apply.) (36)*
    1. patients' response to treatments.
    2. any adverse effects of medications.
    3. the status of their discharge plans.
    4. if the medical diagnosis is correct.
    5. if the patient has any risk factors.
13. The initial assessment is performed on a patient to identify patient problems based on defining characteristics, as well as to identify: *(Select all that apply.) (36)*
    1. risk factors that predispose the patient to developing problems.
    2. responses to a disease process.
    3. adverse effects of drugs.
    4. when patients need assistance to get up in the chair.
    5. what to prescribe for treatment for various disease processes.
14. Important healthcare information that the nurse gathers during the assessment of a patient includes: *(Select all that apply.) (36-37)*

1. vital signs.
2. lung sounds.
3. mobility level.
4. discharge plans.
5. family support.

15. Gordon's Functional Health Patterns Model is an example of what kind of assessment? *(36)*
    1. Body systems approach
    2. Head-to-toe approach
    3. Sociocultural, psychological, spiritual, and developmental approach
    4. High-risk signs and symptoms approach

16. The nurse needs to assess the patient in the hospital for therapeutic effects, side effects, and potential drug interactions during which time? *(36)*
    1. Throughout hospitalization
    2. When the patient has visitors
    3. When the patient requests a PRN medication
    4. While monitoring vital signs

Discuss how nursing diagnosis statements are written.

17. An example of an approved NANDA diagnosis for a patient with a respiratory illness would be: *(Select all that apply.)* *(36)*
    1. Impaired gas exchange.
    2. Impaired verbal communication.
    3. Ineffective airway clearance.
    4. Impaired spontaneous ventilation.
    5. Risk for aspiration.

18. NANDA diagnoses are part of the nursing language that describes: *(Select all that apply.)* *(36)*
    1. syndrome nursing diagnoses.
    2. actual medical diagnoses.
    3. risk/high-risk nursing diagnoses.
    4. wellness nursing diagnoses.
    5. health promotion diagnoses.

19. When writing the nursing diagnosis for medication therapy, the nurse will describe the expected outcomes from the prescribed medications based on the: *(39)*
    1. etiology and contributing factors.
    2. laboratory test results.
    3. recommended routes of the medications.
    4. degree of improvement noted in the symptoms present.

Differentiate between a nursing diagnosis and a medical diagnosis.

20. The nurse analyzes the data collected from the patient assessment to identify signs and symptoms that will be addressed under the nursing diagnosis. These are the: *(37)*
    1. therapeutic intent.
    2. defining characteristics.
    3. measurable outcomes.
    4. contributing factors.

21. When formulating the nursing diagnosis in relation to medications, the nurse will need to identify the: *(39)*
    1. medical diagnosis.
    2. drug monographs.
    3. therapeutic responses.
    4. procedures to ensure patient safety.

22. Two types of nursing diagnoses that apply to all types of medication therapies are: *(44)*
    1. Deficient knowledge and Deficient diversional activity.
    2. Noncompliance and Deficient knowledge.
    3. Risk-prone health behavior and Noncompliance.
    4. Deficient knowledge and Interrupted family processes.

23. The nursing diagnosis differs from the medical diagnosis because the: *(39)*
    1. medical diagnosis identifies defining characteristics.
    2. medical diagnosis identifies alterations in structure and function.
    3. nursing diagnosis identifies alterations in structure and function.
    4. nursing diagnosis identifies a disease or disorder that impairs function.

24. The three components of the nursing diagnosis are: *(40)*
    1. defining characteristics, identified disease process, and contributing factors.
    2. NANDA-approved label, defining characteristics, and contributing factors.
    3. alterations in function, NANDA-approved label, and identified disease process.
    4. defining characteristics, contributing factors, and etiology of the disorder.

Discuss how evidence-based practice is used in planning nursing care.

25. When nurses use evidence-based practice changes for planning nursing care, they are incorporating: *(40)*
    1. tradition.
    2. trial and error.
    3. pilot studies.
    4. validated research.

26. The goal of evidence-based practice is to improve patient outcomes by using: *(41)*
    1. various treatments for medical conditions.
    2. best practices that evolved from research.
    3. the patient's clinical presentation.
    4. prescriptive recommendations of physicians.

27. Discontinuing the use of antiembolism stockings because recent studies have shown them to be ineffective is an example of: *(41)*
    1. nursing intuition.
    2. evidence-based nursing practice.
    3. trial and error.
    4. traditional nursing practice.

28. The four phases of the planning process include: *(Select all that apply.)* **(40)**
    1. setting priorities.
    2. developing measurable goals.
    3. identifying "related to" factors.
    4. formulating nursing interventions.
    5. formulating therapeutic outcomes.

Differentiate between nursing interventions and expected outcome statements.

29. Nursing interventions identify specific nursing actions, while measurable goal statements identify specific: **(41)**
    1. priority settings.
    2. patient behaviors.
    3. changes in patient care needs.
    4. patient responses.
30. It is important for nurses to include the patient and appropriate significant others in decision-making when formulating therapeutic patient outcomes because it will help to: **(42)**
    1. promote cooperation and compliance by the patient.
    2. provide patients with a sense of control over their care.
    3. prepare the patient for evidence-based nursing care.
    4. promote shorter hospital stays.
31. The nurse will identify the therapeutic outcomes of the medications given by: *(Select all that apply.)* **(45)**
    1. reviewing the drug monograph for anticipated effects.
    2. filling out an insurance claim for reimbursement.
    3. identifying the recommended routes of the medications.
    4. determining when laboratory tests need to be scheduled.
    5. identifying the recommended dosage of the medications.

Explain how Maslow's hierarchy of needs is used to prioritize patient needs.

32. Maslow's subcategories of human needs are used in the planning process during the: **(41)**
    1. setting of priorities.
    2. development of measureable goals.
    3. formulation of therapeutic outcomes.
    4. identification of "related to" factors.
33. The five levels of needs identified by Maslow's hierarchy include: *(Select all that apply.)* **(41)**
    1. self-actualization.
    2. safety.
    3. belonging.
    4. physiologic.
    5. priority.
34. Which level of Maslow's hierarchy would be a priority when planning nursing care? **(41)**

    1. Safety needs
    2. Belonging needs
    3. Self-esteem needs
    4. Physiologic needs

Compare and contrast the differences between dependent, interdependent, and independent nursing actions.

35. The nurse is performing a *dependent* nursing action in which scenario? **(42)**
    1. The patient is being monitored for the effects of the medication given at 8 AM.
    2. The patient is being educated on her 8 AM medication by the nurse.
    3. The patient is given her 8 AM medication by the nurse.
    4. The patient is verbalizing that she understands the reasons for the medications she received at 8 AM.
36. The nurse is performing an *interdependent* nursing action in which scenario? **(42)**
    1. The nurse is calling the healthcare provider for pain medication orders.
    2. The nurse is assisting the physical therapist with exercises for the patient.
    3. The nurse is assessing the patient for bowel sounds after surgery.
    4. The nurse is educating the patient in the use of her incentive spirometer.
37. The nurse is performing an *independent* nursing action in which scenarios? *(Select all that apply.)* **(42)**
    1. The patient is being monitored for the effects of the medication given at 8 AM.
    2. The nurse is calling the prescriber for pain medication orders.
    3. The nurse is educating the patient in the use of her incentive spirometer.
    4. The nurse is assessing the patient for bowel sounds after surgery.
    5. The nurse is consulting with dietary services for patient preference for meals.

Discuss how the nursing process applies to pharmacology.

38. The sources that the nurse uses to obtain a medication history include: *(Select all that apply.)* **(44)**
    1. objective data (provided by relatives).
    2. other healthcare professionals.
    3. subjective data (provided by the patient).
    4. drug monographs.
    5. the electronic medical record.
39. When discussing the medication history with a patient, the nurse will ask the patient to identify current medications and drug allergies, as well as: *(Select all that apply.)* **(43)**
    1. diagnostic tests done.
    2. over-the-counter medications used.
    3. food allergies.

4. herbal products used.
5. street drugs used.

40. The nurse can use primary, secondary, and tertiary sources to gain information to complete the medication history. When the nurse obtains vital signs to use as monitoring parameters later, it is considered: *(44)*
    1. a secondary source of information.
    2. a tertiary source of information.
    3. subjective data.
    4. objective data.

41. The medication history that the nurse records includes: *(43)*
    1. current medications and drug allergies.
    2. past medications that are no longer being used and drug allergies.
    3. medications that are prescription-based and drug allergies.
    4. over-the-counter medications and drug allergies.

Patient Education to Promote Health

Answer Key: Textbook page references are provided as a guide for answering these questions. A complete answer key is provided to your instructor.

MATCHING
Match the learning domain on the right with the patient education objective on the left. Domains may be used more than once.

Patient Education Objective

1. _____ demonstrating correct self-administration of insulin

2. _____ requesting more information on adverse effects of a new medication

3. _____ discussing healthcare changes that will occur when discharged, like needing an aide

4. _____ verbalizing the medications needed for pain relief after surgery

Learning Domain

a. cognitive domain
b. affective domain
c. psychomotor domain

REVIEW QUESTIONS

Differentiate among cognitive, affective, and psychomotor learning domains.

5. When the nurse asks the patient to perform a return demonstration of a skill such as injecting insulin or performing a dressing change, the patient is exercising which domain of learning? *(50)*
   1. Affective
   2. Psychomotor
   3. Cognitive
   4. Psychological

6. The affective domain of learning refers to the: *(49)*
   1. thinking portion of the learning process.
   2. learning of a new procedure or skill.
   3. feelings, beliefs, and values that the patient has.
   4. environment that is conducive to learning.

7. The patient has just been instructed on his home-going medications prior to discharge, and the nurse will validate the information that was given by asking the patient to verbalize his understanding. This involves which domain of learning? *(49)*
   1. Cognitive
   2. Affective
   3. Psychomotor
   4. Psychological

Identify the main principles of learning that are applied when teaching a patient, family, or group.

8. When teaching patients and their families, the nurse must recognize the teachable moment. That is when the: *(50)*
   1. nurse starts to ask questions regarding home-going care.
   2. nurse has the time and is ready to start teaching.
   3. patient is gone for a test and the family looks anxious.
   4. patient and/or family start to ask questions.

9. One of the main principles of learning that the nurse incorporates into teaching is that adults learn by: *(50)*
   1. rote memorization.
   2. applying new knowledge to previous learning.
   3. listening to the nurse explain everything.
   4. asking questions.

10. The nurse needs to determine the patient's preferred learning style when educating the patient on continuing care. One way to do this is by using a variety of teaching aids, which may include: *(Select all that apply.) (50)*
    1. pamphlets and charts.
    2. video and motion pictures.
    3. discussing care with the family while the patient is out.
    4. audiocassettes.
    5. smart devices and computer-aided instruction.

Describe the essential elements of patient education in relation to prescribed medications.

11. When the nurse is teaching the patient about her medications, some important considerations can be implemented, such as: *(Select all that apply.)* *(53-54)*
    1. teaching at a time most convenient for the nurse.
    2. determining the patient's readiness to learn.
    3. spacing the content.
    4. organizing the patient education materials.
    5. motivating the patient to learn.
12. During a teaching session that a nurse was having with a patient, the patient suddenly became tearful and turned away. The best response from the nurse at this time is: *(53)*
    1. "Why don't you just read this later, and I can mark you as getting through the material."
    2. "I need to finish this and get it checked off my list, so bear with me."
    3. "I see that you are upset; I can finish this later. Do you want to talk about it?"
    4. "I see that you are not paying attention. Now come on, let's finish this."
13. When teaching older adults about new medications, it is important for the nurse to remember to: *(Select all that apply.)* *(53)*
    1. check for vision or hearing aids.
    2. determine memory impairments.
    3. evaluate gross motor ability.
    4. review content rapidly.
    5. lecture the patient about healthy lifestyles.

Describe the nurse's role in fostering patient responsibility for maintaining well-being and for adhering to the therapeutic regimen.

14. The nurse understands that when teaching a patient and family about lifestyle changes, it is important to: *(Select all that apply.)* *(56)*
    1. tell the patient that she will need to change her lifestyle or else.
    2. keep the content relevant to the patient.
    3. add extra content to further explain points.
    4. remember that learning new ideas may be overwhelming.
    5. keep the patient's wishes in mind.
15. One important aspect of the nurse's role in discussing the patient's medications and adhering to a particular medication regimen is to: *(54)*
    1. adopt a slower pace for teaching younger patients.
    2. dictate to the older adult patient what must be changed.
    3. continue teaching until all content is covered.
    4. repeat the information often, and stop and allow practice.

16. The nurse needs to involve the patient in cooperative goal setting when teaching, which will include: *(Select all that apply.)* *(56)*
    1. what to monitor for.
    2. why prescribed therapy is needed.
    3. when to call the healthcare provider.
    4. where to collect and record essential data.
    5. how to discontinue or alter their medication regimen.

Identify the types of information that should be discussed with the patient or significant others.

17. The nurse is reviewing sources of patient information on the Internet that may be helpful for patients wanting more information after discharge, which include: *(Select all that apply.)* *(55)*
    1. Krames Online.
    2. Therapeutic Choices.
    3. Health on the Net Foundation.
    4. Medline.
    5. CINAHL.
18. Ethnocentric nurses tend to consider patients in the light of the culture: *(54)*
    1. that the patient is from.
    2. that the nurse is from.
    3. of the hospital.
    4. of the home environment.
19. Reasonable expectations that the nurse should have when discussing new treatment therapies include that the: *(56)*
    1. patient will fully understand all instructions.
    2. patient and family will ask appropriate questions and demonstrate adequate understanding of teaching.
    3. family will have to participate in the teaching because most patients are unable to think clearly while in the hospital.
    4. patient will need to be taken care of outside of the hospital, as he will never understand any instructions given.

Discuss specific techniques used in the practice setting to facilitate patient education.

20. The nurse can facilitate appropriate patient teaching by: *(55-56)*
    1. keeping all records of the essential data needed to evaluate the prescribed therapy.
    2. expecting the patient to manage his therapy without further assistance.
    3. contacting the healthcare provider for advice on when to tell the patient to discontinue his medication entirely.
    4. asking the patient to record responses to his medications at home.

21. Which statement by a patient indicates that further teaching is needed? *(56)*
    1. "I will keep a record of my blood pressure the same time of day to see how my medication is working."
    2. "I know that I will need to call my healthcare provider when I start to feel like I did when I came into the hospital."
    3. "I can take my pills when I feel like it, because they can get so expensive."
    4. "I will let my wife know about these pills because she usually helps me remember to take them."

22. When a patient is discharged from the hospital, it is important for the nurse to document: *(57)*
    1. the time the patient left and who accompanied the patient.
    2. all care that was received during hospitalization.
    3. the collaborative problems that will require continued monitoring after discharge.
    4. the nursing diagnoses that were identified on admission.

Principles of Medication Administration and Medication Safety

chapter

6

Answer Key: Textbook page references are provided as a guide for answering these questions. A complete answer key is provided to your instructor.

MATCHING

Match the rights of drug administration on the right with the nursing action on the left. Rights may be used more than once.

Nursing Action

1. _____ triple-checking the drug
2. _____ consult reference book and calculate properly
3. _____ verify the reason for the drug
4. _____ this effects absorption rate
5. _____ check to determine when drug was given last
6. _____ compare exact spelling
7. _____ a major medicolegal consideration
8. _____ ensure two identifiers are used
9. _____ determine appropriate schedule

Seven Rights of Drug Administration

a. right drug
b. right indication
c. right time
d. right dose
e. right patient
f. right route
g. right documentation

REVIEW QUESTIONS

Identify the legal and ethical considerations for medication administration.

10. The rules and regulations established by the state boards of nursing are in place: *(60)*
    1. as guidelines to practice nursing.
    2. to restrict access to healthcare.
    3. when an avoidable complication arises.
    4. to regulate healthcare facilities.
11. Policy statements that are made by nurse practice acts related to medication administration include: *(Select all that apply.)* *(60)*
    1. educational requirements necessary to have prescriptive privileges.
    2. lists of medications that are forbidden to be administered by nurses.
    3. abbreviations approved for use to avoid medication errors.
    4. medications that the nurse can start with IV solutions.
    5. when to claim unfamiliarity with any nursing responsibilities.
12. Prior to any medication administration, the nurse must be able to: *(Select all that apply.)* *(60)*

1. accurately calculate the dose.
2. explain the expected actions of the medication.
3. describe the contraindications for the use of the medication.
4. explain why the medication is ordered.
5. document the patient's response to the medication.

Compare and contrast the various systems used to dispense medications.

13. The floor stock system of dispensing medications used in small hospitals has the advantage of readily available medications, but also has disadvantages such as: *(Select all that apply.)* *(67)*
    1. increased potential for medication errors.
    2. potential misappropriation of medication by hospital personnel.
    3. fewer inpatient prescription orders.
    4. lack of review by a pharmacist for patient order accuracy.
    5. need for larger stocks and frequent drug inventories.
14. The system that provides the advantage of easier inventory control and reduced revenue loss describes the: *(68)*

1. unit-dose system.
2. floor or ward stock system.
3. individual prescription order system.
4. computer-controlled dispensing system.

15. Advantages of the unit-dose system include: *(Select all that apply.)* *(68)*
    1. returned bottles of unused medications are destroyed.
    2. less waste and misappropriation of medications.
    3. quality-control procedures are completed by pharmacists.
    4. packaging that reduces errors.
    5. nurses profile any drug interactions or contraindications.

16. *Pyxis system* refers to what drug dosage system? *(68-69)*
    1. Narcotic inventory system
    2. Individual prescription order system
    3. Unit-dose system used primarily in long-term care
    4. Electronic medication dispensing system

17. The *ward stock system* refers to the: *(67)*
    1. narcotic inventory system.
    2. individual prescription order system.
    3. system used in very small hospitals.
    4. electronic medication dispensing system.

18. The nurse understands that using a computer-controlled ordering and dispensing system means that: *(68-69)*
    1. there is no need to use standard procedures for medications like the Seven Rights.
    2. verification and transcription of medication orders are built into the system.
    3. narcotic inventory will no longer be necessary.
    4. documentation of the patient's response to the medication is not needed.

Identify what a narcotic control system entails.

19. When removing narcotics from a narcotic control system, what must be observed? *(Select all that apply.)* *(70)*
    1. The medications must be passcode-accessible
    2. The date the medication was removed
    3. The time the medication was removed
    4. The name of the nurse who removed the medication
    5. The time the medication was given to the patient

20. A nurse was preparing to administer 3 mg of morphine (a controlled substance) orally to a patient. The medication came in 4 mg/4 mL. What steps must the nurse take when giving this medication? *(Select all that apply.)* *(70)*
    1. Determine the correct amount to give (3 mL).
    2. Ask another nurse to verify the dose and any wasted medication.
    3. Check the time interval since the last dose was given.

4. Complete the controlled substance inventory.
5. Complete the documentation after administration.

21. While checking the narcotics count at the end of a shift, the nurse notes a discrepancy regarding the oral doses of hydromorphone (Dilaudid). What needs to be done next? *(71)*
    1. Security needs to be called.
    2. The nurse manager needs to be notified.
    3. The patients' charts need to be reviewed for proper documentation.
    4. An appropriate interval of time must be observed before any narcotics can be removed.

Define the four categories of medication orders.

22. What type of drug order indicates that nurses are to administer the medication for a specific number of doses? *(73)*
    1. Stat orders
    2. Verbal orders
    3. Single orders
    4. Standing orders

23. The nurse is reviewing an order that states "nifedipine 30 mg SL now." This is an example of what type of order? *(73)*
    1. Stat order
    2. Verbal order
    3. Single order
    4. Standing order

24. When should PRN medications be administered? *(73)*
    1. When the patient asks for some.
    2. When the nurse determines a medication is warranted and can be safely administered.
    3. When the healthcare provider orders it.
    4. When the appropriate time interval has elapsed.

25. When does the drug prescribed using the term *stat* need to be given? *(72-73)*
    1. At the next opportunity the nurse has to administer the medication.
    2. Immediately and one time only.
    3. When the patient asks for it.
    4. Immediately and at scheduled time intervals.

Identify common types of medication errors and the actions that can be taken to prevent them.

26. The nurse is preparing to administer a patient's 8 AM medications and notes that the dosage for the drug raloxifene (Evista) is outside the normal range. What will the nurse need to do next? *(75)*
    1. Verify the dosage with the healthcare provider.
    2. Notify the pharmacy that the drug dose is in error.
    3. Administer the medication and report the error.
    4. Refuse to administer all of the patient's medications until the error is corrected.

27. Medication errors that the nurse could make when administering a drug include: *(Select all that apply.)* *(73)*

1. omission (missed dose).
2. duplication (extra dose given).
3. inventory.
4. formatting.
5. wrong time.

28. Technology is being used to help prevent medication errors by: *(Select all that apply.)* **(74)**
    1. robotics to administer medications to free up nurses.
    2. automatic delivery of medications.
    3. computerized provider order entry.
    4. smart pumps for controlled administration.
    5. barcoded administration.

29. After administering a dose of the oral antihistamine fexofenadine (Allegra), the nurse noticed the patient had already received a dose 2 hours before. This type of error refers to a(n): **(74)**
    1. prescribing error.
    2. administration error.
    3. monitoring error.
    4. transcription error.

30. During the administration of a medication, the patient asks the nurse why the medication has been ordered. The nurse will respond with the answer, which is part of which one of the Seven Rights? **(76)**
    1. Right patient
    2. Right route
    3. Right dosage
    4. Right indication

31. When preparing to administer a medication to a patient, the nurse is not able to verify that the medication order is appropriate. What actions does the nurse take? *(Select all that apply.)* **(75)**
    1. Documents the reasons for refusal to administer the drug in accordance with the policies of the employing institution.
    2. Contacts the person who prescribed the drug.
    3. If the prescriber cannot be contacted, notifies the nursing supervisor on duty.
    4. Administers the medication because it went through pharmacy, and they would have caught a problem if there was one.
    5. Informs the patient about the disagreement with the treatment prescribed.

Identify precautions used to ensure the right drug is prepared and given to the right patient.

32. The nurse was preparing to administer a dose of the antibiotic cefepime (Maxipime). Place the steps in the order that the nurse will follow to ensure the right drug is administered. **(75-76)**
    1. _____ Document the drug.
    2. _____ Triple-check that the drug name and dose are correct prior to administration.
    3. _____ Identify the patient using two patient identifiers.

4. _____ Administer the medication via the correct route.
5. _____ Check the order.

33. Medication reconciliation is a process that is designed to reduce medication errors and involves which steps? *(Select all that apply.)* **(74)**
    1. Developing a list of current medications being taken by the patient
    2. Comparing the lists of current medications with prescribed ones
    3. Developing a list of prescribed medications
    4. Reviewing potential adverse drug events
    5. Comparing written blanket orders

34. The healthcare provider has written an order after the patient returns from angiography that states "Resume all preprocedure medications." This is known as: **(74)**
    1. a handoff order.
    2. medication reconciliation.
    3. a blanket order.
    4. a redundant order.

List the seven rights of medication administration.

35. After the nurse has administered an appropriate dose of a medication that has been ordered, the nurse must now: **(78)**
    1. scan the medication into the barcode system.
    2. notify the prescriber that the medication has been administered.
    3. chart in the medication administration record the date and time given.
    4. review the order and perform triple-checks.

36. When reconstituting a medication to be administered, the nurse needs to clearly label it with the: *(Select all that apply.)* **(78)**
    1. patient's name.
    2. dose.
    3. concentration.
    4. amount to be discarded.
    5. name of the nurse.

37. What is the most effective method the nurse uses for identifying a pediatric patient for medication administration? **(77)**
    1. Asking the child his or her name.
    2. Asking a family member the child's name.
    3. Checking the child's identification bracelet.
    4. Checking the room number with the bed the child is in.

Identify the appropriate nursing documentation of medications including the effectiveness of each medication.

38. Examples of what the nurse will need to document to identify how effective medications are include: *(Select all that apply.)* **(78)**
    1. questions the family asks about home-going medications.

2. noting any nausea and vomiting prior to oral medications.
3. monitoring vital signs.
4. checking blood sugar prior to insulin administration.
5. specific assessments such as lung sounds.

39. When determining the therapeutic effectiveness of a medication, the nurse will: *(79)*
    1. ask the patient to repeat the name of the medication.
    2. call the healthcare provider to verify each medication ordered.
    3. notify the pharmacist regarding the patient's response.
    4. document the patient's response and notify the healthcare provider when appropriate.

40. The nurse gave an antiemetic medication 30 minutes ago and is checking on the patient to determine the effectiveness. Which scenario indicates the medication worked? *(79)*
    1. The patient states that he feels much better and his pain is all gone.
    2. The patient states he feels a lot less nauseated.
    3. The patient states he is starting to feel dizzy and lightheaded.
    4. The patient states that he is feeling weaker and getting chills.

Percutaneous Administration

chapter

7

Answer Key: Textbook page references are provided as a guide for answering these questions. A complete answer key is provided to your instructor.

MATCHING
Match the dose form on the right with the application site on the left. More than one dose form may be used for the application sites.

Application Site

1. _____ ear
2. _____ eye
3. _____ skin
4. _____ mucous membranes
5. _____ buccal cavity

Dose Form

a. powders
b. aqueous solutions
c. transdermal patches
d. creams
e. ointments
f. buccal tablets

REVIEW QUESTIONS

Identify the equipment needed and the techniques used to apply each of the topical forms of medications to the skin.

6. The factors affecting the absorption of topical medications include the: *(Select all that apply.)* *(81)*
   1. concentration of the medication.
   2. length of time the medication is in contact with the skin.
   3. patient's personal hygiene preferences.
   4. thickness and hydration of the skin.
   5. size and depth of the skin area affected.

7. The major advantages of the percutaneous route for medication administration include: *(Select all that apply.)* *(81)*
   1. there is a long duration of action and reapplication is often not required.
   2. it allows for limited exposure of the medication to a specific site of application.
   3. improved patient personal hygiene measures.
   4. decrease in systemic adverse effects.
   5. reduces the spread of infection.

8. The percutaneous route of medication administration includes which forms of application? *(Select all that apply.)* *(81)*
   1. Eyedrops
   2. Rectal suppositories
   3. Nasal sprays
   4. Inhaled nebulized medications
   5. Subcutaneous injections

9. Why is it important for the nurse to wear gloves when applying a topical ointment or transdermal patch? *(82)*
   1. So the correct amount of medication is applied to the patient's skin.
   2. To identify a patient's sensitivity to contact materials.
   3. To avoid inadvertent absorption of the medication by the nurse through the skin.
   4. So the dose is not contaminated with the nurse's skin cells.

10. List the steps in the order in which the nurse would apply a medicated lotion to a patient. *(82)*
    1. _____ Apply lotion firmly but gently by dabbing the surface.
    2. _____ Perform hand hygiene and apply gloves.
    3. _____ Document the application.
    4. _____ Shake the suspension well for a uniform appearance of the lotion.
    5. _____ Clean the area and the equipment used, and make sure that the patient is comfortable.

11. What is important for the nurse to remember when applying ointment to patient's skin? *(Select all that apply.)* *(82)*
    1. Ointments are semisolid preparations of medicinal substances in an oily base.
    2. Ointments are to be applied directly to the skin or mucous membranes.

3. Ointments must be reapplied frequently because they are absorbed easily.
4. The use of ointments helps to keep the medication in prolonged contact with the skin.
5. Ointments generally cannot be removed easily with water.

Describe the purpose of and the procedure used for performing patch testing.

12. The purpose of patch testing is to identify: *(83)*
    1. when a patient will need an antiemetic.
    2. which area of the patient's skin is sensitive to topical ointments.
    3. which antibiotic will be effective against an infection.
    4. specific sensitivity the patient has to allergens.
13. The nurse is preparing to apply a patch test to a patient, and the patient asks what he will need to remember after leaving the clinic. The nurse will respond: *(83)*
    1. "You will need to call the clinic in 48 hours if you have a reaction."
    2. "You will need to report back to the clinic after a week and we will read the results."
    3. "You will not be able to shower for a week while the patch test is on your back."
    4. "You will need to return to the clinic to have the test read in 48 hours."
14. Common areas on the body that are used during a patch test include: *(Select all that apply.) (83)*
    1. face.
    2. thighs.
    3. back.
    4. neck.
    5. arms.
15. Commonly used symbols for reading reactions to allergen testing include: *(Select all that apply.) (85)*
    1. ## (2#) (only erythema noted).
    2. ++ (2+) (2- to 3-mm wheal with flare).
    3. ++++ (4+) (> 5-mm wheal).
    4. – – – (3–) (no wheal response).
    5. +++ (3+) (3- to 5-mm wheal with flare).
16. The nurse is working in an allergy clinic. What should be taken into consideration by the nurse when administering allergy testing to patients? *(Select all that apply.) (84)*
    1. Ensuring that emergency equipment is in the immediate area in case of an anaphylactic response
    2. Positioning the patient so that the surface where the test material is to be applied is horizontal
    3. Administering antihistamine and antiinflammatory agents immediately before the test
    4. Cleansing the area where the allergens are to be applied with an alcohol wipe and allowing the area to dry before starting testing
    5. Documenting "no reaction" at the control site on the patient's chart

17. In addition to documenting the date, time, drug name, dose, and site of administration of the patch test, the nurse needs to document: *(85)*
    1. any signs and symptoms of adverse effects.
    2. when the patient bathed or showered last.
    3. the number of patch test kits available.
    4. when hand hygiene was performed.

Identify the equipment needed, the sites and techniques used, and the patient education required when nitroglycerin ointment is prescribed.

18. List in the correct order the steps the nurse will use to administer nitroglycerin ointment. *(85-86)*
    1. _____ Position patient to expose surface to be used, and remove applicator paper from previous dose.
    2. _____ Apply dose to patient's skin and cover with plastic wrap or tape.
    3. _____ Perform hand hygiene and don gloves.
    4. _____ Gather nitroglycerin ointment, applicator paper, and nonallergenic adhesive tape.
    5. _____ Squeeze proper amount of nitroglycerin ointment onto applicator paper.
19. The nurse is applying a nitroglycerin transdermal disk and expects the disk to be applied: *(87)*
    1. every 12 hours.
    2. every day.
    3. every 7 days.
    4. every 3 days.
20. After applying a nitroglycerin transdermal disk, the nurse will educate the patient about: *(87)*
    1. the number of times the disks can be reused.
    2. documentation needed.
    3. how and when to apply the disks.
    4. never wearing the disks while showering.
21. The nurse will identify the expected effectiveness of the nitroglycerin ointment when the patient states she has had: *(86)*
    1. a severe drop in blood pressure and lightheadedness.
    2. an increase in angina attacks.
    3. relief from angina attacks.
    4. itching and a rash with the drug.
22. Documentation of the application of nitroglycerin ointment should include: *(Select all that apply.) (86)*
    1. date, time, dosage, site, route of administration, and nurse's name.
    2. patient assessments such as blood pressure, pulse, and pain relief.
    3. signs and symptoms of adverse drug effects.
    4. essential patient education that was reviewed.
    5. any family present in the room at the time.
23. The nurse was completing the process of administering 1 inch of nitroglycerin ointment to the patient's left chest; the proper documentation will include the date and: *(86)*

1. 0915, nitroglycerin ointment (1") to chest, Nancy Nurse.
2. 0915, 1" nitroglycerin ointment applied to left chest, topical, Nancy Nurse.
3. 0915, nitroglycerin ointment, Nancy Nurse.
4. 0915, 1" nitroglycerin ointment, topical, Nancy Nurse.

Identify the equipment needed, the sites and techniques used, and the patient education required when transdermal medication systems are prescribed.

24. Patient education for transdermal medication systems includes what to do when: *(Select all that apply.)* *(87)*
    1. documenting the administration of the medication.
    2. taking a shower.
    3. the disk becomes loose.
    4. a drug-free period of time is prescribed.
    5. disposing of the medication.
25. When administering nitroglycerin percutaneously to a patient, what does the nurse do? *(86)*
    1. Performs hand hygiene and wears gloves.
    2. Applies wax paper over the site of the nitroglycerin to enhance absorption of the drug.
    3. Ensures that the drug is on the patient 24 hours a day, 7 days a week to avoid complications.
    4. Always places the nitroglycerin ointment over the left chest to provide the most effective route of drug delivery to the heart.
26. The common sites used for application of any transdermal medication disks include: *(Select all that apply.)* *(87)*
    1. chest.
    2. face.
    3. flank.
    4. upper arms.
    5. axilla.
27. The nurse is reviewing an order to administer a topical powder to a patient. What should the nurse know prior to administration? *(88)*
    1. The site of application, the indication for the medication, and the expected effects.
    2. The site of application, the common adverse effects of the medication, and the family's expectations.
    3. The site of application, the intended purpose of the medication, and the patient's usual sleep pattern.
    4. The site of application, the patient's bathing preference, and the expected effects.
28. Proper administration of powdered medications includes: *(88)*
    1. performing hand hygiene before and after administration; gloves are not necessary.
    2. shaking the container prior to administration to evenly distribute the medication.

3. applying the powder to wet skin to allow it to "cake" on.
4. applying the powder over the area using a thick layer.

29. An important point to consider when administering powdered medication is: *(88)*
    1. how long it needs to stay on.
    2. when to wash it off.
    3. where to apply it.
    4. which medication will wear off faster.

Describe the dose forms, the sites and equipment used, and the techniques for the administration of medications to the mucous membranes.

30. List in order the steps the nurse will take to administer eyedrops. *(90)*
    1. _____ Hold the eyelid open and approach the eye from below with the medication dropper or tube of ointment.
    2. _____ Discard gloves, perform hand hygiene, and document.
    3. _____ Position the patient so that the back of the head is firmly supported on a pillow and the face is directed toward the ceiling.
    4. _____ Obtain the prescribed bottle or tube of eye medication.
    5. _____ Perform hand hygiene and don gloves.
31. The proper technique used to administer eyedrops or eye ointment is to ask the patient to look: *(90)*
    1. down and pull up on the lower eyelid.
    2. up and pull up on the lower eyelid.
    3. up and pull down on the lower eyelid.
    4. down and pull down on the lower eyelid.
32. Medications that can be applied to mucous membranes are available in which dose forms? *(Select all that apply.)* *(88)*
    1. Sublingual
    2. Gel
    3. Tablet
    4. Liquid
    5. Capsule

Compare the techniques that are used to administer eardrops to patients who are less than 3 years old with those that are used for patients who are 3 years and older.

33. When administering eardrops to a child younger than 3 years, the nurse should restrain the child, turn the head to the appropriate side, and gently pull the earlobe: *(91)*
    1. downward and back.
    2. downward and forward.
    3. upward and back.
    4. upward and forward.
34 The nurse is explaining to the mother of a 2-year-old child how to administer eardrops to her child, and

the mother asks if cotton can be placed in the ear after administration. The nurse responds: *(91)*
1. "Yes, that is recommended. Let me show you how."
2. "No, that practice is not accepted anymore."
3. "Yes, we can use a cotton-tipped applicator and insert it as far back as it will go."
4. "No, the healthcare provider will frown on that."

35. When applying eardrops to a child, the nurse notices that there is a large amount of wax buildup in the ear canal. What will the nurse do next? *(91)*
    1. Call the healthcare provider and ask for another route for the medication to be administered.
    2. Administer the medication, as the wax will not be a problem.
    3. Remove the wax with a cotton-tipped applicator prior to administration.
    4. Obtain an order to gently remove wax by irrigating the ear canal prior to administration.

Describe the purpose, the precautions necessary, and the patient education required for those patients who require medications via inhalation.

36. Which types of medications are available in the oral inhalation dose form? *(Select all that apply.)* *(94)*
    1. Bronchodilators
    2. Fentanyl
    3. Nitroglycerin
    4. Corticosteroids
    5. Allergens

37. Bronchodilators and corticosteroids may be administered by oral inhalation through the mouth using an aerosolized, pressurized: *(95)*
    1. semisolid emulsion.
    2. buccal tablet.
    3. metered-dose inhaler (MDI).
    4. oral drop/oral spray.

38. When administering medications via the inhalation route, the nurse instructs the patient to: *(Select all that apply.)* *(95-96)*
    1. inhale deeply over 10 seconds after activating the MDI.
    2. shake the medication canister before using MDIs.
    3. rinse his or her mouth after using an inhaled corticosteroid.
    4. blow into the dry powder inhaler (DPI).
    5. place one end of the extender in the mouth and close the lips around it.

Identify the equipment needed, the site, and the specific techniques required to administer vaginal medications or douches.

39. List in order the steps the nurse takes to administer a vaginal suppository. *(97)*
    1. _____ Perform hand hygiene and don gloves.
    2. _____ Lubricate the gloved index finger and insert the suppository.
    3. _____ Ask the patient to void prior to administration.
    4. _____ Place the patient in the correct position and unwrap a vaginal suppository that has been warmed to room temperature, and lubricate it with a water-soluble lubricant.
    5. _____ Document the administration.

40. The nurse is instructing the patient to be positioned for a vaginal medication, and asks the patient to lay on her: *(97)*
    1. left side.
    2. back with legs in the air.
    3. stomach with knees tucked.
    4. back in the lithotomy position.

41. Douching is recommended for which use? *(97)*
    1. When there is a vaginal infection present.
    2. As a normal feminine hygiene practice.
    3. After a vaginal suppository has been administered.
    4. As an effective method of birth control.

Enteral Administration

chapter

8

Answer Key: Textbook page references are provided as a guide for answering these questions. A complete answer key is provided to your instructor.

MATCHING

Match the term on the right with the definition on the left.

Definition		Term
1. _____ medication dissolved in a concentrated solution of sugar and water		a. tablet
2. _____ medication dissolved in alcohol and water		b. capsule
3. _____ small, cylindrical gelatin containers that hold dry powder or liquid medication		c. lozenge
4. _____ dry powdered medication compressed into small disks		d. elixir
5. _____ liquids with solid insoluble drug particles dispersed solution, requires shaking prior to use		e. emulsion
6. _____ flat disks in a sugar base form to dissolve slowly in the mouth		f. syrup
7. _____ dispersion of small droplets of water in oil by means of an emulsifying agent		g. suspension

REVIEW QUESTIONS

Describe general principles of administering solid forms of oral medications.

8. The *enteral* route refers to medications administered directly into the gastrointestinal (GI) tract, which includes: *(Select all that apply.)* *(100)*
   1. rectally.
   2. sublingually.
   3. percutaneous endoscopic gastrostomy (PEG) or G tube.
   4. orally.
   5. nasogastric (NG) tube.
9. The advantages of the oral route of medication administration include being: *(Select all that apply.)* *(100)*
   1. easy to administer.
   2. easy to retrieve if given in error.
   3. slow absorption rate.
   4. convenient.
   5. economical.
10. When administering a solid form of medication to a patient, which procedures does the nurse apply? *(Select all that apply.)* *(105)*
    1. Using a tablet-crushing device for appropriate medications when patients have difficulty swallowing.

2. Having the patient place the medication on the front of the tongue.
3. Encouraging the patient to keep the head back while swallowing.
4. Remaining with the patient while the medication is being taken.
5. Having the patient drink a full glass of water with the medication.

Compare the different techniques that are used with a unit-dose distribution system and an electronic controlled distribution system.

11. Which system requires the nurse to use a security access code and password? *(104)*
    1. Medication administration record system
    2. Electronic controlled system
    3. Medication card system
    4. Unit-dose distribution system
12. When distributing medications via the computer-controlled system, the nurse will need to verify the medication using: *(104)*
    1. the medication profile.
    2. another nurse to verify the correct dosage.
    3. the patient to correctly identify the medication.
    4. a medication card.

13. Which system is designed to allow the nurse to hand the medication to the patient and allow him or her to read the package label? *(104)*
    1. Computer-controlled system
    2. Medication administration record
    3. Medication card system
    4. Unit-dose system

Identify general principles used for liquid-form oral medication administration.

14. To read the correct amount of a liquid medication that has been poured into a medicine cup, the nurse reads the meniscus, which is the: *(106)*
    1. lowest point of the convex curve in the cup.
    2. highest point of the concave curve in the cup.
    3. lowest point of the concave curve in the cup.
    4. highest point of the convex curve in the cup.
15. The term for small droplets of water in oil or oil in water that are used to mask bitter tastes or provide better solubility to certain drugs is: *(102)*
    1. elixir.
    2. suspension.
    3. syrup.
    4. emulsion.
16. When administering a liquid form of an oral medication to an infant, the nurse confirms that the: *(107)*
    1. infant is alert.
    2. infant is positioned so that the head is lowered.
    3. syringe or dropper is at the tip of the infant's tongue.
    4. medicine is given rapidly to facilitate swallowing of the medicine.

Cite the equipment needed, techniques used, and precautions necessary when administering medications via a nasogastric tube.

17. The alternative route of giving medications by NG is generally done because the patient: *(Select all that apply.)* *(107)*
    1. refuses to take medications orally.
    2. is unable to swallow.
    3. has had gastric surgery.
    4. has a disorder of the esophagus.
    5. is comatose.
18. List in order the proper procedure for administration of a drug via an NG tube. *(109)*
    1. _____ Clamp the tubing at the end of medication administration.
    2. _____ Position the patient upright and check the location of the NG tube.
    3. _____ Flush the tube with 30 mL of air using a larger syringe.
    4. _____ Perform hand hygiene and don gloves.
    5. _____ Document the medication and how the patient tolerated the procedure.

19. Why should the nurse flush the NG tube after administration of enteral formulas? *(Select all that apply.)* *(110)*
    1. To allow better absorption of the formula from the stomach.
    2. To ensure the tube stays in position after the feeding.
    3. To maintain the patency of the tube.
    4. To prevent the formula remaining in the tube from supporting bacterial growth.
    5. To remove the formula from the tubing.
20. When working with patients receiving enteral feedings via a gastrostomy tube, the nurse performs which actions? *(Select all that apply.)* *(110)*
    1. Checks the residual volume before each feeding
    2. Checks to ensure the presence of bowel sounds
    3. Checks the position of the tube to ensure that it is still in the stomach
    4. Discards unused portions of feedings every 8 hours
    5. Changes the administration equipment every 12 hours

Cite the equipment needed and the technique required when administering rectal suppositories and disposable enemas.

21. What instructions will the nurse give the patient when administering a rectal suppository? *(111)*
    1. "Hold your breath while I insert the suppository."
    2. "Get out of bed as soon as I get the suppository in place."
    3. "Try to hold the suppository for 15 to 20 minutes."
    4. "You will need to lay on your right side before I can insert this suppository."
22. Rectal suppositories are those medications that the nurse will be able to: *(111)*
    1. have the patient self-administer.
    2. ask another nurse to give, as it is not pleasant to do.
    3. discard if a suppository becomes soft.
    4. administer when the patient is lying on the left side.

23. List in order the procedure for administration of a disposable enema. *(112)*

    1. _____ Check pertinent patient monitoring parameters (i.e., last time defecated).

    2. _____ Explain carefully to the patient the procedure for administering an enema.

    3. _____ Put on gloves, remove protective covering from the rectal tube, and lubricate.

    4. _____ Position the patient on the left side, and drape.

    5. _____ Remove and discard gloves, and wash hands thoroughly.

24. When administering an enema to an adult, what does the nurse do? *(112)*

    1. Encourages the patient to hold the solution for about 5 minutes before defecating.

    2. Tells the patient not to flush the toilet until the nurse returns and can see the results of the enema.

    3. Inserts 1 inch of the lubricated rectal tube into the rectum.

    4. Heats the enema to 101° F to ensure comfort in administration.

Parenteral Administration: Safe Preparation of Parenteral Medications

chapter

9

Answer Key: Textbook page references are provided as a guide for answering these questions. A complete answer key is provided to your instructor.

MATCHING
Match the syringe on the right with the volume of medication on the left.

Volume of Medication		Syringe	
1. _____	tuberculin syringe	a.	½ mL
2. _____	1-mL syringe	b.	7.5 mL
3. _____	3-mL syringe	c.	0.04 mL
4. _____	5-mL syringe	d.	3.5 mL
5. _____	10-mL syringe	e.	2 mL

REVIEW QUESTIONS

Identify the parts of a syringe and needle, as well as examples of the safety-type syringes and needles.

6. The outer portion of the syringe on which the calibrations for the measurements of drug volume are located is called the: *(116)*
   1. gauge.
   2. barrel.
   3. tip.
   4. plunger.
7. The inner cylindrical portion of the syringe that fits snugly into the barrel is called the: *(116)*
   1. gauge.
   2. barrel.
   3. tip.
   4. plunger.
8. The portion of the syringe that holds the needle is called the: *(116)*
   1. gauge.
   2. barrel.
   3. tip.
   4. plunger.
9. The difference between a safety syringe and an ordinary syringe is that the safety syringe has an attachment called a: *(122)*
   1. sleeve or sheath.
   2. needle cover.
   3. calibration measure.
   4. plunger topper.

Describe how to select the correct needle gauge and length and how the needle gauge is determined.

10. The gauge of the needle is marked on the hub of the needle and on the outside of the disposable package, and the nurse knows this number represents the: *(120)*
    1. maximum volume allowed when using this needle.
    2. length of the needle.
    3. inner diameter of the needle.
    4. actual dose the needle can hold.
11. An example of the gauge and length of a needle used for intradermal injection is: *(121)*
    1. 25 gauge; 5/8 inch.
    2. 18 gauge; 1 inch.
    3. 29 gauge; 3/8 inch.
    4. 20 gauge; 1/2 inch.
12. The proper needle gauge is usually selected based on the viscosity (thickness) of the solution to be injected and the: *(120)*
    1. site of injection.
    2. dose of the medication.
    3. barrel of the syringe.
    4. calibration scale used.
13. Low-dose insulin syringes are used to measures doses of insulin up to: *(117-118)*
    1. 100 units.
    2. 50 units.
    3. 25 units.
    4. 10 units.
14. The nurse is instructing the patient on the use of the insulin pen and includes in the teaching: *(Select all that apply.) (118)*
    1. how to hold the pen correctly.
    2. how to dial in the correct amount of insulin.
    3. when the cartridge needs to be replaced.
    4. that once the needle is attached, it is left attached until all of the insulin is used.
    5. which site to insert the needle and inject the proper dose.

List the advantages and disadvantages of using a glass syringe versus a plastic syringe.

15. What is one difference between glass syringes and plastic ones, when reading the volumes within the syringes? *(116)*
    1. Glass syringes read volumes at the calibration scale, parallel to the plunger.
    2. Glass syringes read volumes at the calibration scale, parallel to the rubber flange.
    3. Plastic syringes read volumes at the calibration scale, parallel to the tip of the rubber flange.
    4. Plastic syringes read volumes at the calibration scale, below the level of the plunger.

16. Plastic syringes use which scales for calibration? *(116)*
    1. Millimeter scale
    2. Liter scale
    3. Milligram scale
    4. Milliliter scale

17. What are the two types of syringe tips that can be found on plastic syringes? *(116)*
    1. Catheter tip and locking tip
    2. Reverse tip and outer flange
    3. Collar tip and non-collar tip
    4. Male tapered end tip and threaded locking collar tip

Compare and contrast the volumes of medications that can be measured in a tuberculin syringe and those of larger-volume syringes.

18. The nurse is preparing to give a subcutaneous injection of 0.5 mL of dalteparin. The medication should be injected using a: *(118)*
    1. standard plastic syringe.
    2. tuberculin syringe.
    3. prefilled syringe.
    4. glass syringe.

19. The nurse knows that the use of the tuberculin syringe is limited to: *(117-118)*
    1. tuberculin inoculations.
    2. volumes smaller than 1 mL.
    3. insulin administration.
    4. volumes greater than 1 mL.

20. Insulin syringes are specifically calibrated to measure: *(117-118)*
    1. epinephrine doses.
    2. any volume smaller than 1 mL.
    3. tuberculin inoculations.
    4. insulin doses.

Compare and contrast the advantages and disadvantages of using prefilled syringes.

21. The *advantages* of using a prefilled syringe include the: *(Select all that apply.)* *(118)*
    1. syringe is used once and discarded.
    2. time that is saved in preparing a standard amount of medication for one injection.
    3. nurse can expect these syringes are cheaper than multi-vials.

4. chance for contamination of the syringe is decreased.
5. use of a cartridge to hold the prefilled syringe.

22. The *disadvantages* of using a prefilled syringe include the: *(Select all that apply.)* *(118)*
    1. nurse does not draw up the medication.
    2. limitation that a second medication generally cannot be added to the cartridge.
    3. syringe is used once and discarded.
    4. use of a cartridge to hold the prefilled syringe.
    5. expense of using a prefilled syringe.

23. Many hospital pharmacies will use prefilled syringes for specific doses of medication for some patients; for example: *(Select all that apply.)* *(118-119)*
    1. Carpuject syringes.
    2. insulin pen.
    3. glass syringes.
    4. tuberculin syringes.
    5. EpiPen.

24. The nurse was preparing to administer an intramuscular (IM) injection of 1 mg of Haldol, which was in a concentration of 1 mg/1 mL, to a confused patient. In the medication room, the nurse was choosing the correct needle and syringe from the shelf. The patient was an adult of normal weight, so the nurse picked: *(120-121)*
    1. 25 gauge, 5/8-inch needle, with a 5-mL syringe.
    2. 21 gauge, 1 1/2-inch needle, with a 3-mL syringe.
    3. 29 gauge, 3/8-inch needle, with a 10-mL syringe.
    4. 23 gauge, 1-inch needle, with a 1-mL syringe.

25. Two nurses were in the medication room discussing the difference between the volume of medication that can be given in any subcutaneous site and the intradermal site. Which statement is correct? *(121)*
    1. "I always give between 0.5 mL and 1 mL for intradermal, and less than 0.1 mL for subcutaneous injections."
    2. "I always give between 0.01 mL and 0.1 mL for intradermal, and less than 1 mL for subcutaneous injections."
    3. "I always give between 0.01 mL and 0.1 mL for intradermal, and less than 2 mL for subcutaneous injections."
    4. "I always give between 0.1 mL and 1 mL for intradermal, and less than 0.5 mL for subcutaneous injections."

26. Which route is commonly thought to be fast for absorption of medication? *(115)*
    1. Oral
    2. Intradermal
    3. Rectal
    4. Intramuscular

Differentiate among ampules, vials, and Mix-O-Vials.

27. Glass containers that may be scored or have a darkened ring around the neck and usually contain a single dose of a medication are called: *(124)*
    1. rubber diaphragm vials.
    2. metal lid vials.
    3. Mix-O-Vials.
    4. ampules.

28. Glass or plastic containers that contain one or more doses of a sterile medication are called: *(124)*
    1. vials.
    2. scored ampules.
    3. Mix-O-Vials.
    4. ringed ampules.

29. How does the nurse use a Mix-O-Vial? (A single dose of medication is normally contained in the Mix-O-Vial.) *(127-128)*
    1. By applying pressure to the rubber stopper between the two chambers.
    2. By applying pressure to the top rubber diaphragm plunger.
    3. By shaking the upper chamber (which contains the solvent) until it falls into the lower chamber (which contains the drug).
    4. By shaking the lower chamber (which contains the drug) until the upper chamber (which contains the solvent) falls down into the lower chamber.

Describe the technique used to prepare two different drugs in one syringe (e.g., insulin).

30. When administering NPH and Regular insulin together in the same syringe, what does the nurse do? *(129)*
    1. Discards NPH insulin if it is cloudy.
    2. First injects the amount of air equal to the amount of insulin to be withdrawn into the Regular insulin.

    3. First draws up the NPH insulin to be administered.
    4. Is careful not to inject any of the first type of insulin already in the syringe into the vial.

31. The nurse is preparing to administer 58 units of insulin and knows that which is true regarding insulin syringes? *(Select all that apply.)* *(118, 129)*
    1. The shorter lines on the Regular insulin syringe represent 2 units measured.
    2. The longer lines on the low-dose insulin syringe measure 10 units of insulin.
    3. The low-dose insulin syringe can be used for this dose.
    4. The longer lines on the Regular insulin syringe measure 10 units of insulin.
    5. The shorter lines on the low-dose insulin syringe represent 2 units measured.

32. List in order the correct sequence the nurse will follow to mix NPH and Regular insulin. *(129)*
    1. _____ Insert the needle into the NPH vial, withdraw the correct amount of insulin.
    2. _____ Inject air into the Regular vial and invert the bottle and withdraw the correct volume of Regular insulin.
    3. _____ Fill the syringe with air to an amount equal to the correct amount of NPH, insert the needle into the vial, inject air, remove needle.
    4. _____ Check the insulin order and wipe the tops of both vials of insulin.
    5. _____ Fill the syringe with air to an amount equal to the correct amount of Regular insulin.

Parenteral Administration: Intradermal, Subcutaneous, and Intramuscular Routes

chapter 10

Answer Key: Textbook page references are provided as a guide for answering these questions. A complete answer key is provided to your instructor.

MATCHING

Match the description on the right with the intramuscular site on the left.

Intramuscular Site	Description
1. _____ vastus lateralis	a. Considered easiest site when patients are sitting
2. _____ ventrogluteal	b. Considered easiest site for self-administration
3. _____ rectus femoris	c. Considered the preferred IM site for infants
4. _____ deltoid	d. Considered easiest site when patients are side-lying

REVIEW QUESTIONS

Describe the technique that is used to administer a medication via the intradermal route.

5. The most common site for the administration of intradermal medication is the inner aspect of which body part? *(132)*
   1. thigh
   2. forearm
   3. upper arm
   4. shin

6. When administering intradermal allergy testing for a patient, which steps does the nurse perform? *(Select all that apply.) (132-134)*
   1. Asks the patient if he or she has taken any antihistamine or antiinflammatory agents for 24–48 hours before the test
   2. Uses an alcohol wipe to clean the skin
   3. Injects the volume ordered, usually 0.01 to 0.05 mL, into the subcutaneous tissue
   4. Aspirates for blood once the needle has been inserted
   5. Wipes the site with alcohol after injection

7. When preparing to provide allergy testing to a patient using the intradermal injection technique, what does the nurse do? *(133-134)*
   1. Inserts the needle at a 90-degree angle with the needle bevel facing down
   2. Recaps the needle used before disposing of it in a puncture-resistant container
   3. Wears gloves
   4. Deposits the solution being injected into the subcutaneous tissue under the skin

List the equipment needed, and describe the technique that is used to administer a medication via the subcutaneous route.

8. The nurse is teaching a patient about the importance of rotating subcutaneous insulin injection sites. Which statement made by the patient indicates a need for additional teaching? *(135)*
   1. "Common subcutaneous sites for administering insulin include upper arms, anterior thighs, and the abdomen."
   2. "The fastest site of absorption is when I inject into the abdomen."
   3. "I need to rotate injection sites to prevent lipohypertrophy, which will slow insulin absorption."
   4. "Exercise will not affect the rate of insulin absorption."

9. Which route of injection is considered the fastest for medication absorption? *(136)*
   1. Intradermal
   2. Intraocular
   3. Subcutaneous
   4. Intramuscular

10. The nurse was educating a patient about heparin injections that would need to be continued at home, and the patient states: "I know that I need to inject my abdominal area just under the skin, right?" How should the nurse respond? *(135)*
    1. "That's correct, this is an intradermal injection."
    2. "Actually, this injection will go into the subcutaneous tissue, or the fat that is under the skin."

3. "Well, this injection is designed to be delivered into your muscle, so instead of the abdomen, you will give it in your leg."
4. "That is almost correct. It will go under your skin, but not in your abdomen; it will be in your arm."

Describe the technique used to administer medications intramuscularly.

11. The nurse is preparing to administer an IM injection in the ventrogluteal area. What does the nurse do first? *(136-137)*
    1. Positions the patient supine with the toes pointed outward.
    2. Has the patient flex the gluteal muscle to minimize pain from the injection.
    3. Identifies the site by forming a "V" on the greater trochanter of the femur.
    4. Holds the syringe at a 30-degree angle to the surface of the patient's skin.
12. List the steps in order that the nurse will follow to administer an IM injection. *(138-139)*
    1. _____ Apply a small bandage to the site.
    2. _____ Explain carefully to the patient what will be done.
    3. _____ Insert the needle at the correct angle and depth for the site being used.
    4. _____ Carefully identify the patient using two patient identifiers.
    5. _____ Provide for privacy; position the patient appropriately.
13. The most important instruction to follow for the nurse administering an IM injection is to: *(138-139)*
    1. add a bubble of air to the syringe.
    2. pinch the skin into a bunch prior to injection.
    3. tell the patient to hold his breath during the injection.
    4. correctly identify the patient prior to administration.

Describe the landmarks that are used to identify the vastus lateralis muscle, the rectus femoris muscle, the ventrogluteal area, and the deltoid muscle before medication is administered.

14. When administering an IM injection in the deltoid muscle, the nurse will locate the site: *(138-139)*
    1. one hands-breadth below the greater trochanter.
    2. by palpating the top of the shoulder and measuring down three finger-breadths.
    3. with the needle directed slightly upward toward the crest of the ilium.
    4. on the anterior lateral thigh.
15. This site for injection is located by placing the palm of the hand on the lateral portion of the greater trochanter, the thumb pointing toward the groin, the index finger on the anterior superior iliac spine, and the middle finger extended to the iliac crest. *(137-138)*
    1. rectus femoris muscle
    2. deltoid muscle
    3. vastus lateralis muscle
    4. ventrogluteal muscle
16. The vastus lateralis muscle is located: *(136-137)*
    1. in the buttock area.
    2. below the shoulder.
    3. on the thigh.
    4. under the armpit.

Identify suitable sites for the intramuscular administration of medication in an infant, a child, an adult, and an older adult.

17. The nurse knows that the best site for an IM injection for an infant is the: *(137)*
    1. rectus femoris muscle.
    2. deltoid muscle.
    3. vastus lateralis muscle.
    4. ventrogluteal muscle.
18. The nurse is planning to administer an IM injection for an adult patient who needs a flu vaccine (0.5 mL). Which muscle is the best to use? *(138-139)*
    1. Rectus femoris muscle
    2. Deltoid muscle
    3. Vastus lateralis muscle
    4. Ventrogluteal muscle
19. Prior to administering an IM injection into an older adult, the nurse: *(Select all that apply.) (138-139)*
    1. checks the patient's allergy list.
    2. asks another nurse to verify the correct dose prior to administration.
    3. verifies two patient identifiers.
    4. cleanses the skin with an alcohol wipe.
    5. inserts the needle to a depth of 1/2 inch and injects the medication.

Parenteral Administration: Intravenous Route

chapter

11

Answer Key: Textbook page references are provided as a guide for answering these questions. A complete answer key is provided to your instructor.

MATCHING

Match the definition on the right with the complication on the left.

	Complication		Definition
1. _____	extravasation	a.	symptoms include dyspnea, cough, coarse crackles, and frothy sputum
2. _____	infiltration	b.	pathogens from a local infection invade the bloodstream causing fever and chills
3. _____	speed shock	c.	an inflammation of a vein
4. _____	thrombophlebitis	d.	the leakage of an intravenous solution into the surrounding tissue
5. _____	pulmonary edema	e.	redness, warmth, purulent drainage, swelling, and burning pain along the course of the vein
6. _____	septicemia	f.	the leakage of an irritating chemical into the surrounding tissue
7. _____	localized infection	g.	an inflammation of a vein with an associated blood clot
8. _____	phlebitis	h.	flushing, tightness in the chest, and hypotension

REVIEW QUESTIONS

Define intravenous (IV) therapy and describe the three intravascular compartments.

9. The three types of vessels that comprise the intravascular compartment are the: *(144)*
   1. interstitial spaces, extracellular spaces, and intracellular spaces.
   2. arteries, veins, and capillaries.
   3. sinuses, cavities, and pleural spaces.
   4. arterioles, alveoli, and veins.

10. The nurse is preparing to administer an antibiotic IV and knows that the advantages of intravenous medications are: *(Select all that apply.)* *(144)*
    1. this route is more comfortable than subcutaneous.
    2. the patient tends to be less mobile.
    3. large volumes of fluids can be rapidly administered.
    4. medications can be directly injected into the vein.
    5. the possibility of infection is higher via this route.

11. The spontaneous movement of water from an area of low electrolyte concentration to an area of high electrolyte concentration refers to a phenomenon that creates: *(150)*
    1. equilibrium.
    2. osmotic pressure.
    3. electrolyte and protein compartments.
    4. hydraulic pressure.

Discuss the different IV access devices used for IV therapy.

12. What types of needles are used to access an implanted port? *(149)*
    1. Huber needles
    2. Subclavian needles
    3. Hickman needles
    4. Intravenous needles

13. The nurse prepares to start an IV on a patient and is gathering the supplies needed, which include: *(Select all that apply.)* *(157)*
    1. sterile gloves.
    2. alcohol wipes.
    3. tourniquet.
    4. transparent dressing.
    5. IV catheter.

14. In calculating IV fluid rates, microdrip chambers form how many drops per milliliter? *(144)*
    1. 10
    2. 15

3. 20
4. 60

15. Common locations of peripheral IVs include the: *(Select all that apply.)* *(152)*
    1. metacarpal vein.
    2. dorsal vein.
    3. jugular vein.
    4. basilic vein.
    5. cephalic vein.
16. When a patient needs long-term IV or home IV therapy, the various types of catheters used will be: *(Select all that apply.)* *(153)*
    1. peripheral.
    2. central venous.
    3. implantable access device.
    4. midline catheter.
    5. Hickman or Broviac catheter.
17. Peripherally inserted central catheter (PICC) lines are inserted into the: *(148)*
    1. jugular vein and threaded down to end at the superior vena cava.
    2. cephalic vein and threaded down to end at the superior vena cava.
    3. subclavian vein and threaded down to end at the superior vena cava.
    4. metacarpal vein and threaded down to end at the superior vena cava.

Differentiate between isotonic, hypotonic, and hypertonic IV solutions and explain their clinical uses.

18. A patient has been admitted to the healthcare facility after experiencing a GI bleed at home, which has now resolved. The patient now has an intravascular fluid volume deficit. Which IV fluid does the nurse anticipate will be ordered for the patient? *(150)*
    1. 0.9% sodium chloride
    2. 0.2% sodium chloride
    3. 0.45% sodium chloride
    4. 5% dextrose in water
19. Hypertonic solutions (e.g., parenteral nutrition solutions) are administered through central infusion lines directly into the: *(151)*
    1. inferior vena cava.
    2. jugular veins.
    3. peripheral veins.
    4. superior vena cava.
20. Which type of solution contains fewer electrolytes and more free water? *(151)*
    1. Isotonic
    2. Hypotonic
    3. Hypertonic
    4. Replacement solutions

Identify the general principles for administering medications via the IV route.

21. IV administration dose forms are available in: *(Select all that apply.)* *(152)*

1. vials.
2. prefilled syringes.
3. ampules.
4. large-volume IV solution bags.
5. tablets.

22. In general, what does the nurse need to consider regarding any medication administered via the IV route? *(Select all that apply.)* *(153-154)*
    1. How far the needle is inserted into the vein.
    2. The purpose of the drug.
    3. How fast the drug should be administered.
    4. Whether the drug should be administered in a central vein or a peripheral vein.
    5. That an armboard will need to be used for all IV fluids.
23. The types of sites for IV administration include: *(Select all that apply.)* *(147)*
    1. central venous catheters.
    2. peripheral venous catheters.
    3. midline catheters.
    4. PICCs.
    5. arterial catheters.

Compare and contrast the differences between a peripheral IV line and a central IV line.

24. An example of a peripheral IV access device is a: *(Select all that apply.)* *(147)*
    1. butterfly needle.
    2. scalp needle.
    3. large-bore needle.
    4. winged needle.
    5. Huber needle.
25. The nurse was teaching a patient about the need for a central IV access device and recognized further teaching was needed when the patient stated: *(148-149)*
    1. "I guess my veins in my arms are shot from the repeated IVs I have had, so a central line makes sense."
    2. "Since I will need to have long-term antibiotic therapy, it makes sense to have a PICC line."
    3. "I understand about Port-a-Caths since my wife's cousin had one for her chemotherapy."
    4. "As I understand it, this will mean that I will need to have my PICC changed every 3 months."
26. The advantages of a peripheral IV line over a central IV line include that the peripheral line: *(Select all that apply.)* *(148)*
    1. has fewer complications than the central line.
    2. is easier to insert than the central line.
    3. lasts longer than the central line.
    4. costs less than the central line.
    5. requires fewer assessments than the central line.

Describe the correct techniques for administering medications by means of a saline lock, an IV bag, an infusion pump, and a secondary piggyback set.

27. The nurse follows which steps when administering a medication by a saline lock? *(Select all that apply.)* **(160-161)**
    1. Selects a syringe several milliliters larger than that required by the volume of the drug.
    2. After determining that the IV has a blood return, injects saline for the flush followed by the medication at the rate specified by the manufacturer.
    3. After the medication is administered, inserts another syringe containing normal saline to flush the remaining drug from the catheter.
    4. Maintains constant pressure on the plunger of the syringe used to flush the line after the medication has been administered while simultaneously withdrawing the needle from the injection port to prevent backflow of blood.
    5. Verifies the saline dose with another qualified nurse.

28. The nurse is hanging a bag of normal saline for a patient who has been diagnosed with dehydration and notices that the peripheral IV that was placed in the patient's hand has become dislodged. What should the nurse do next? **(172)**
    1. Advance the catheter into the vein.
    2. Resecure the catheter to the patient's hand.
    3. Remove the catheter and insert another one.
    4. Use the catheter, as it should migrate back into place.

29. While inserting an IV into a patient, the nurse has applied a tourniquet to help locate a vein. What other techniques are used in conjunction with a tourniquet to dilate the vein? *(Select all that apply.)* **(158-159)**
    1. Place the extremity in a dependent position.
    2. Apply cool, moist towels.
    3. Have the patient open and close his or her hand repeatedly.
    4. Apply a heating pad.
    5. Massage the vein.

Describe the recommended guidelines and procedures for IV catheter care.

30. Which statements about PICCs are correct? *(Select all that apply.)* **(148)**
    1. They are not available for pediatric use.
    2. PICC line insertion is only attempted in the operating room.
    3. PICC lines are easier to maintain than short peripheral catheters because the incidence of infiltration and phlebitis is less frequent.
    4. They should not be used for long-term administration of total parenteral nutrition.
    5. It is necessary to flush the PICC line with a saline-heparin solution after every use, or daily if not used.

31. When providing care to a patient receiving IV therapy, which actions does the nurse perform? *(Select all that apply.)* **(170)**
    1. Wears gloves to inspect the IV site
    2. Applies topical antibiotic ointment to the insertion site
    3. If it appears that the IV access device is clotted, attempts to clear the needle by flushing with fluid
    4. Checks the drip chamber; if it is less than half full, squeezes it to fill more completely
    5. Checks the temperature of the solution being infused because cold solutions can cause spasms in the vein

32. A patient has been ordered a PICC for the administration of medications. The nurse has taught the patient about the insertion procedure, use, and care of the PICC line. Which statement made by the patient indicates a need for further teaching? **(148)**
    1. "I will be placed under general anesthesia to have this intravenous line inserted."
    2. "I will be able to go home with a PICC line."
    3. "My PICC line can last up to a year if it is properly cared for."
    4. "The PICC line should be flushed with a saline-heparin solution after every use, or daily if not used."

Identify baseline assessments for IV therapy and proper maintenance of patency of IV lines and implanted access devices.

33. List in order the steps the student nurse will take while administering a medication via saline lock to a patient after hand hygiene was performed and the patient identified. **(160)**
    1. _____ Flushes the lock with saline while observing the IV site at the catheter tip for swelling and monitors for reports of discomfort.
    2. _____ Wipes the injection cap with an alcohol wipe for 15 seconds.
    3. _____ Injects the medication at the proper rate, followed by saline for a flush.
    4. _____ Documents the date, time, drug, dosage, rate of administration, assessment data, and how well the procedure was tolerated.
    5. _____ Accesses the injection portal with a syringe containing flush solution and gently pulls back on the plunger for a blood return.

34. Which statements about implantable infusion ports are correct? *(Select all that apply.)* **(149)**
    1. Blood products can be administered through an implantable infusion port.
    2. One port of a two-port system may be reserved for drawing blood samples.
    3. An implanted central venous access catheter may remain in place for over a year and only requires a saline-heparin solution flush after every access or once monthly.

4. The CDC recommends that central venous catheters be routinely replaced to prevent catheter-related infection.
5. The infusion port can accommodate up to 100 punctures before it needs to be changed.

35. Important assessments to perform for IV therapy include determining when the IV needs to: *(Select all that apply.)* **(169-170)**
    1. be documented regarding the IV insertion site according to agency policy.
    2. be flushed or determine the patency of the IV with fluids running.
    3. have the dressing changed on the site.
    4. be changed to another insertion site according to agency policy.
    5. provide blood draws for labs.

Explain the signs, symptoms, and treatment of the complications associated with IV therapy (e.g., phlebitis, thrombophlebitis, localized infection, septicemia, infiltration, extravasation, air in tubing, pulmonary edema, catheter embolism, and "speed shock").

36. The nurse will monitor the patient with an IV for signs and symptoms of the inflammation of a vein, called: **(170)**
    1. extravasation.
    2. thrombus.
    3. phlebitis.
    4. thrombophlebitis.

37. The complication of extravasation is important to monitor in patients with IV drug drips and medications given IV push because this may mean that: **(171)**
    1. the patient will experience warmth, tenderness, swelling, and burning pain in the IV site.
    2. the needle tip has punctured the vein.
    3. the patient is now becoming infected.
    4. serious tissue damage may occur.

38. The nurse recognizes circulatory overload in a patient experiencing which symptoms while receiving IV therapy? **(172)**
    1. Dyspnea, cough, anxiety, rhonchi, and possible cardiac dysrhythmias
    2. Engorged neck veins; dyspnea; reduced urine output; edema; bounding pulse; and shallow, rapid respirations
    3. A blood clot that breaks loose, traveling to the lungs
    4. Dyspnea, pleuritic pain, sweating, tachycardia, cough, and cyanosis

Drugs That Affect the Autonomic Nervous System

Answer Key: Textbook page references are provided as a guide for answering these questions. A complete answer key is provided to your instructor.

MATCHING

Match the sympathetic or parasympathetic nervous system on the right with the action on the left. Insert "a" for sympathetic or "b" for parasympathetic.

Actions

1. _____ relaxation of the GI sphincters
2. _____ dilation of the pupil in the eye (mydriasis)
3. _____ relaxation of the bronchial muscles
4. _____ constriction of the systemic veins
5. _____ constriction of the bronchial muscles
6. _____ constriction of the pupil in the eye (miosis)
7. _____ constriction of the GI sphincters

Sympathetic or Parasympathetic Nervous System

a. Sympathetic or adrenergic receptors
b. Parasympathetic or cholinergic receptors

REVIEW QUESTIONS

Scenario: A 69-year-old male was admitted to the hospital with an exacerbation of his asthma. He has a history of hypertension, diabetes, and benign prostatic hyperplasia.

Describe how the central nervous system differs from the peripheral nervous system.

8. The primary difference between the central nervous system (CNS) and the peripheral nervous system (PNS) is the: *(175)*
   1. CNS controls the autonomic nervous system, while the PNS controls the motor nervous system.
   2. CNS is comprised of afferent and efferent nerves, while the PNS is comprised of the brain and the spinal cord.
   3. CNS controls all involuntary movements and the PNS controls all voluntary movements.
   4. CNS is comprised of the brain and the spinal cord, while the PNS is comprised of afferent and efferent nerves.

9. The PNS is further subdivided into the somatic nervous system that controls voluntary movement and the: *(175)*
   1. vascular system.
   2. autonomic nervous system.
   3. system of neurotransmitters.
   4. endocrine system.

10. What primary function is controlled by the motor nervous system? *(175)*
    1. Secretion of enzymes into the digestive system
    2. Skeletal muscle contractions
    3. Involuntary contraction of the digestive system
    4. Transmission of neuronal impulses within the synaptic junctions

11. Once the neurotransmitter has been released into the synaptic junction, what happens? *(176)*
    1. A message is transmitted down the axon to the nerve fibers.
    2. A decrease in response to nerve stimulation occurs.
    3. Postsynaptic receptors are stimulated by the neurotransmitter.
    4. Symptoms of Parkinson's disease become apparent.

12. Neurotransmitters that are released into synapses at the end of neurons are able to: *(Select all that apply.)* *(176)*
    1. respond by secreting another neurotransmitter.
    2. stimulate the next neuron.
    3. stimulate receptors on an end organ.
    4. inhibit electrical impulses through the neuron.
    5. secrete an enzyme.
13. Examples of end-organ receptors that are part of the nervous system and are usually at the end of the nerve chain are: *(Select all that apply.)* *(176)*
    1. adrenal glands.
    2. heart muscle.
    3. brain.
    4. smooth muscles of the GI tract.
    5. spinal cord.

Name the most common neurotransmitters known to affect central nervous system function and identify the two major neurotransmitters of the autonomic nervous system.

14. The major types of receptors found in the autonomic nervous system include: *(Select all that apply.)* *(176)*
    1. alpha.
    2. beta.
    3. dopaminergic.
    4. gamma.
    5. delta.
15. The nerve endings that liberate acetylcholine are called: *(176)*
    1. adrenergic fibers.
    2. cholinergic fibers.
    3. cholinergic agents.
    4. adrenergic agents.
16. The nurse understands that the two major neurotransmitters of the autonomic nervous system are: *(176)*
    1. norepinephrine and acetylcholine.
    2. epinephrine and acetylcholine.
    3. epinephrine and dopamine.
    4. norepinephrine and epinephrine.
17. Which system controls blood pressure and body temperature? *(176)*
    1. Motor nervous system
    2. Voluntary nervous system
    3. Autonomic nervous system
    4. Somatic nervous system

Explain how drugs inhibit the actions of cholinergic and adrenergic fibers.

18. Medications that cause effects similar to those produced by the adrenergic neurotransmitter norepinephrine are called: *(176)*
    1. adrenergic agents.
    2. cholinergic agents.
    3. anticholinergic agents.
    4. adrenergic-blocking agents.

19. Medications used to inhibit the effects of the natural neurotransmitter acetylcholine secreted by cholinergic fibers are called: *(176)*
    1. adrenergic agents.
    2. cholinergic agents.
    3. anticholinergic agents.
    4. adrenergic-blocking agents.
20. Medications used to inhibit the effects of the natural catecholamines secreted by the adrenergic fibers are called: *(176)*
    1. adrenergic agents.
    2. cholinergic agents.
    3. anticholinergic agents.
    4. adrenergic-blocking agents.
21. Cholinergic fibers are those nerve endings that secrete which neurotransmitter? *(176)*
    1. Histamine
    2. Acetylcholine
    3. Dopamine
    4. Norepinephrine

Identify two broad classes of drugs used to stimulate the adrenergic nervous system.

22. Since the cholinergic agents and the adrenergic agents have opposite effects, the medications that slow down heart rates and cause pupillary constriction are: *(182)*
    1. cholinergic agents.
    2. adrenergic-blocking agents.
    3. anticholinergic agents.
    4. adrenergic agents.
23. The class of drugs that has the opposite effect of the cholinergic agents and causes pupillary dilation and rapid heart rate is: *(176-177)*
    1. cholinergic agents.
    2. adrenergic-blocking agents.
    3. anticholinergic agents.
    4. adrenergic agents.
24. Adrenergic fibers are those nerve endings that secrete which neurotransmitter? *(176)*
    1. Histamine
    2. Acetylcholine
    3. Dopamine
    4. Norepinephrine
25. The body's catecholamines that are produced primarily from nerve terminals; the adrenal medulla; and selected sites in the brain, kidneys, and GI tract include: *(176)*
    1. dopamine, glycine, and gamma-aminobutyric acid.
    2. norepinephrine, epinephrine, and dopamine.
    3. prostaglandins, histamine, and cyclic adenosine monophosphate (cAMP).
    4. enkephalins, endorphins, and histamine.
26. The catecholamines that are secreted naturally in the body include: *(Select all that apply.)* *(176)*
    1. dopamine.
    2. acetylcholine.

3. epinephrine.
4. serotonin.
5. norepinephrine.

Review the actions of adrenergic agents and the conditions that require the use of these drugs.

27. A nurse was reviewing the order for albuterol (Proventil, Ventolin), an adrenergic agent used for the patient in the scenario, and remembered that the effects of this agent on diabetics can cause: *(178)*
    1. hypotension.
    2. allergic reactions.
    3. hyperglycemia.
    4. hypoglycemia.
28. A patient in the scenario experiences orthostatic hypotension as a result of taking an adrenergic-blocking agent for treatment of hypertension. Which measures does the nurse incorporate into this patient's plan of care? *(Select all that apply.)* *(183)*
    1. Monitor blood pressure in the standing position daily.
    2. Monitor blood pressure daily in the supine position.
    3. Teach the patient to rise slowly from a supine or sitting position.
    4. Encourage the patient to sit down if feeling faint.
    5. Discontinue the adrenergic-blocking agent.
29. Stimulation of the adrenergic receptors causes smooth muscle of the bronchial tree to relax, which results in: *(176)*
    1. stridor.
    2. wheezing.
    3. bronchodilation.
    4. bronchoconstriction.

Describe the benefits of using beta-adrenergic blocking agents for hypertension, angina pectoris, cardiac dysrhythmias, and hyperthyroidism.

30. Stimulation of beta$_2$ receptors in a patient results in which assessment findings? *(Select all that apply.)* *(176-177)*
    1. Bronchoconstriction
    2. Uterine relaxation
    3. Bronchodilation
    4. Tachycardia
    5. Orthostatic hypotension
31. Which medication is the preferred treatment for the patient in the scenario with asthma in need of treatment with a beta blocker? *(179)*
    1. Propranolol
    2. Timolol
    3. Nadolol
    4. Atenolol
32. What are serious adverse effects of beta-adrenergic blocking agent therapy? *(Select all that apply.)* *(182)*
    1. Bradycardia
    2. Wheezing
    3. Orthopnea

4. Hypoglycemia
5. Nausea

Identify diseases in which beta-adrenergic blocking agents should not be used, and discuss why they should not be used.

33. Beta-adrenergic blocking agents such as carvedilol (Coreg) must be used with caution in diabetic patients because these agents may induce, as well as mask, the signs of: *(182)*
    1. tachycardia.
    2. hypoglycemia.
    3. hyperglycemia.
    4. wheezing.
34. The nurse understands a possible effect of administering beta blockers to the patient in the scenario with a known respiratory disease such as asthma is: *(180)*
    1. wheezing.
    2. bronchodilation.
    3. bronchoconstriction.
    4. stridor.
35. Since beta-adrenergic blocking agents have the potential to cause hypotension, bradycardia, and heart failure, it is important to monitor for symptoms of heart failure including an increase in: *(Select all that apply.)* *(180)*
    1. edema.
    2. crackles.
    3. urinary retention.
    4. hypoglycemia.
    5. dyspnea.

Describe clinical uses and the predictable adverse effects of cholinergic agents and anticholinergic agents.

36. Patients with which condition would most likely benefit from the dopaminergic effects of adrenergic agents? *(177)*
    1. Parkinson's disease
    2. Guillain-Barré syndrome
    3. Amyotrophic lateral sclerosis
    4. Multiple sclerosis
37. For patients who have benign prostatic hyperplasia and difficulty voiding, the drugs that help by increasing contractions of the urinary bladder are from which class of drugs? *(182)*
    1. Anticholinergic agents
    2. Adrenergic agents
    3. Cholinergic agents
    4. Adrenergic-blocking agents
38. Anticholinergic agents are used clinically in the treatment of which disorders? *(Select all that apply.)* *(183)*
    1. Tachycardia
    2. Bradycardia
    3. Orthostatic hypotension
    4. Ophthalmic disorders
    5. GI motility disorders

Student Name_____ Date_____

Drugs Used for Sleep

Answer Key: Textbook page references are provided as a guide for answering these questions. A complete answer key is provided to your instructor.

MATCHING

Match the drug classification on the right with the drug name on the left. Classifications may be used more than once.

Drug Name

1. _____ diphenhydramine (Benadryl)
2. _____ triazolam (Halcion)
3. _____ lorazepam (Ativan)
4. _____ secobarbital (Seconal)
5. _____ zolpidem (Ambien)
6. _____ pentobarbital (Nembutal)
7. _____ temazepam (Restoril)

Drug Classification

a. barbiturates
b. benzodiazepines
c. nonbarbiturates, nonbenzodiazepines

REVIEW QUESTIONS

Scenario: A nurse was taking care of a 58-year-old patient who complained of not being able to sleep. To understand the exact problem, the nurse asked the patient if she was having trouble getting to sleep or if she woke up during the night and could not get back to sleep.

Differentiate among the terms *sedative* and *hypnotic*; *initial*, *intermittent*, and *terminal insomnia*; and *rebound sleep* and *paradoxical excitement*.

8. The nurse's questions to the patient in the scenario are intended to determine if there is which type of insomnia? *(188)*
   1. Initial insomnia or rebound insomnia
   2. Initial insomnia or intermittent insomnia
   3. Initial insomnia or terminal insomnia
   4. Initial insomnia or transient insomnia
9. The nurse knows that sedatives are drugs that can be used for patients complaining of insomnia. Barbiturates are one of the classes of sedatives that are not commonly prescribed because they may cause: *(190)*
   1. paradoxical excitement.
   2. terminal insomnia.
   3. rebound insomnia.
   4. paradoxical depression.
10. The phrase *rebound sleep* refers to the: *(188)*

   1. increase in amount of REM sleep that causes restlessness and vivid nightmares.
   2. return of normal sleep patterns after a hypnotic is discontinued.
   3. return to previous insomnia symptoms.
   4. decrease in the amount of REM sleep that causes increased drowsiness.
11. After discussing with the patient in the scenario the best drugs to use for insomnia, the nurse recognized the need for further education when the patient stated: *(188-190)*
   1. "So you are saying that I should take drugs for my insomnia for short periods of time to prevent the side effects."
   2. "I see; if I use a hypnotic prior to going to bed this will help with my insomnia."
   3. "You are right. If I don't start getting better sleep it will start to interfere with my work."
   4. "So you are saying that the best type of drug to use for insomnia is a sedative."
12. *Insomnia* is best defined as: *(188)*
   1. getting fewer than 5 hours of sleep a night.
   2. the inability to sleep.
   3. episodes of REM sleep that last only a few minutes.
   4. experiencing a drifting or floating sensation.

Identify alterations found in the sleep pattern when hypnotics are discontinued.

13. The nurse was teaching a patient about the use of hypnotics and what to expect when they are discontinued. Which is a correct statement? *(188)*
    1. "You should avoid the unpleasant consequences of rebound sleep and stay on the medication prescribed."
    2. "Sedatives have the same effect as hypnotic medications."
    3. "Insomnia is not a disease, but a symptom of physical or mental stress. Your problem will continue after you no longer take the sleeping pill."
    4. "Habitual use of benzodiazepines does not ever result in physical dependence."

14. Which medications and/or substances does the nurse identify as potentially inducing or aggravating insomnia? *(Select all that apply.)* *(189)*
    1. Benzodiazepines
    2. Anticonvulsants
    3. Caffeine
    4. Nicotine
    5. Alcohol

15. After long-term administration of sedative-hypnotic agents, the patient may experience what if the medications are discontinued? *(Select all that apply.)* *(188)*
    1. Severe REM rebound sleep
    2. Restlessness
    3. Recurrent insomnia
    4. Drowsiness
    5. Quick return of normal sleep patterns

Cite nursing interventions that can be implemented as an alternative to administering a sedative-hypnotic medication.

16. While teaching patients about nonpharmacologic methods to enhance sleep, which statement does the nurse include? *(190)*
    1. "Do not go to bed at the same time each night; go to bed when you feel the most tired."
    2. "Eat your heaviest meal of the day about 45 minutes before you plan to go to bed."
    3. "Exercise during the day, not near bedtime."
    4. "Avoid drinking milk before going to bed."

17. The nurse knows that the patient who has complained of insomnia can benefit from some alternative methods of inducing sleep such as: *(Select all that apply.)* *(189-190)*
    1. limit stimulants close to bedtime.
    2. avoid heavy meals late in the evening.
    3. be sure to exercise within 30 minutes of bedtime.
    4. substitute decaffeinated beverages close to bedtime.
    5. try warm milk and crackers as a bedtime snack.

18. The nurse was reviewing a diet choice made by a patient who was suffering from insomnia. Which

choice would be a good alternative to a sedative? *(189)*
    1. Hot black tea and a cookie before bed
    2. Chocolate bar and hot milk
    3. Glass of wine and dark chocolate
    4. Herbal tea and crackers

Compare the effects of barbiturates and benzodiazepines on the central nervous system.

19. Which statements does the nurse include when teaching a patient about zolpidem (Ambien) therapy? *(197)*
    1. "Daytime drowsiness is generally not a problem with this medication."
    2. "If you have difficulty sleeping, increase the dose by one-half."
    3. "No physical dependency will develop with use of this drug."
    4. "Take the medication about 3 hours before you plan on going to sleep."

20. Benzodiazepines work by: *(192)*
    1. suppressing REM and stages III and IV sleep patterns.
    2. stimulating the neurotransmitter dopamine that initiates sleep.
    3. binding to receptors that stimulate the release of gamma-aminobutyric acid (GABA).
    4. activating the sleep function of the cerebral cortex.

21. The use of barbiturates has declined because of the adverse effects of: *(190)*
    1. a long half-life that causes residual daytime sedation.
    2. ultra–short-acting agents that affect the tolerance to the drug.
    3. short-acting agents that cause rebound insomnia.
    4. an increase in bizarre dreams.

Identify the antidote drug used for the management of benzodiazepine overdose.

22. The therapeutic outcomes of benzodiazepine therapy include: *(Select all that apply.)* *(193)*
    1. preoperative sedation with amnesia.
    2. short-term use to produce sleep.
    3. mild sedation.
    4. management of migraines.
    5. increased amount of REM sleep.

23. A nurse was caring for a 54-year-old patient who was admitted for benzodiazepine overdose after taking over 20 lorazepam (Ativan) tablets. The nurse expects which medication to be ordered for the treatment of the overdose? *(193)*
    1. Quazepam (Doral)
    2. Flumazenil (Romazicon)
    3. Triazolam (Halcion)
    4. Butabarbital (Butisol)

24. Rapid discontinuance of benzodiazepines after long-term use may result in symptoms similar to those of alcohol withdrawal, such as: *(Select all that apply.)* **(193)**
    1. headaches.
    2. weakness.
    3. anxiety.
    4. grand mal seizures.
    5. delirium.

Identify laboratory tests that should be monitored when benzodiazepines or barbiturates are administered for an extended period.

25. Since one of the common adverse effects of benzodiazepines is blood dyscrasias, the nurse will monitor which lab values? *(Select all that apply.)* **(195)**
    1. Platelets
    2. Red blood cells
    3. Electrolytes
    4. White blood cells with differential
    5. Prothrombin time

26. The symptoms of hepatotoxicity are anorexia, nausea, vomiting, jaundice, hepatomegaly, splenomegaly, and abnormal liver function tests such as: *(Select all that apply.)* **(195)**
    1. bilirubin.
    2. platelets.
    3. aspartate aminotransferase [AST].
    4. alanine aminotransferase [ALT].
    5. alkaline phosphatase.

27. A pregnancy test may be ordered when a patient is started on a benzodiazepine because: **(195)**
    1. withdrawal symptoms are worse for pregnant mothers.
    2. of an increased incidence of maternal deaths after use of the drugs.
    3. of an increased incidence of birth defects, because these agents cross the placenta.
    4. these agents cross into breast milk.

Drugs Used for Parkinson's Disease

chapter

14

Answer Key: Textbook page references are provided as a guide for answering these questions. A complete answer key is provided to your instructor.

MATCHING

Match the drug classification on the right with the drug name on the left. Classifications may be used more than once.

Drug Name

1. _____ entacapone
2. _____ carbidopa
3. _____ selegiline
4. _____ apomorphine
5. _____ pramipexole
6. _____ rasagiline

Drug Classification

a. monoamine oxidase inhibitors type B
b. dopamine agonists
c. nonergot dopamine agonists
d. COMT inhibitors

REVIEW QUESTIONS

Scenario: A 57-year-old patient who was diagnosed with Parkinson's disease is admitted to an inpatient unit to regulate his medications.

Identify the signs and symptoms of Parkinson's disease.

7. The nurse caring for the patient in the scenario expects to see the patient exhibit symptoms that include difficulty walking and possibly stooped posture, as well as: *(Select all that apply.)* *(200)*
   1. muscle tremors.
   2. muscle weakness with rigidity.
   3. posture and equilibrium changes.
   4. slowness of movement in performing daily activities.
   5. labile emotions.
8. Parkinson's disease is caused by a deterioration of the: *(200)*
   1. levodopa receptors.
   2. dopaminergic neurons.
   3. cholinergic fibers.
   4. acetylcholine neurons.
9. Although Parkinson's disease is primarily considered a disease that affects the patient's ability to walk, it also has nonmotor symptoms such as: *(Select all that apply.)* *(200)*
   1. orthostatic hypotension.

   2. nocturnal sleep disturbances.
   3. nausea and vomiting.
   4. daytime somnolence.
   5. bladder incontinence.
10. This classification of drugs used to treat parkinsonism by reducing the metabolism of dopamine in the brain is: *(205)*
    1. anticholinergic agents.
    2. monoamine oxidase type B inhibitors.
    3. COMT inhibitors.
    4. selective serotonin reuptake inhibitors.
11. Which agents are used in the treatment of Parkinson's disease primarily because they provide symptomatic relief from excessive acetylcholine? *(202)*
    1. Monoamine oxidase type B inhibitors
    2. Selective serotonin reuptake inhibitors
    3. Anticholinergic agents
    4. Dopamine agonists
12. The symptom of Parkinson's disease manifested as extremely slow body movements that may eventually progress to a total lack of movement is known as: *(204)*
    1. propulsive movement.
    2. dyskinesia.
    3. bradykinesia.
    4. akinesia.

Identify the neurotransmitter that is found in excess and the neurotransmitter that is deficient in people with parkinsonism.

13. With Parkinson's disease, which neurotransmitter is deficient? *(215)*
    1. Norepinephrine
    2. Dopamine
    3. Serotonin
    4. Acetylcholine

14. The neurotransmitter that is considered to be in excess in Parkinson's disease is: *(215)*
    1. serotonin.
    2. norepinephrine.
    3. acetylcholine.
    4. dopamine.

15. What can be a cause of secondary parkinsonism? *(Select all that apply.) (200-201)*
    1. Hereditary
    2. Intracranial infections
    3. Head trauma
    4. Tumors
    5. Unknown causes

Describe the reasonable expectations of the medications that are prescribed for the treatment of Parkinson's disease.

16. The goal of treatment for Parkinson's disease is to: *(Select all that apply.) (202)*
    1. moderate the symptoms of the disease.
    2. slow the progression of the disease.
    3. speed up the absorption of dopamine.
    4. slow the deterioration of acetylcholine.
    5. cure the disease.

17. Which statement does the nurse include when teaching a patient with Parkinson's disease about the drug apomorphine (Apokyn)? *(210)*
    1. It is chemically related to morphine, but does not have any opioid activity.
    2. It is used to treat hypermobility associated with the "weaning off" of dopamine agonists.
    3. It is administered intravenously.
    4. It commonly causes hypertension in patients who initially start therapy with this drug.

18. Which medication used in treating patients with Parkinson's disease reduces the destruction of dopamine in the peripheral tissues, allowing significantly more dopamine to reach the brain to eliminate the symptoms of parkinsonism? *(214)*
    1. Entacapone (Comtan)
    2. Ropinirole (Requip)
    3. Apomorphine (Apokyn)
    4. Selegiline (Eldepryl)

19. Generally, patients with Parkinson's disease will be treated with carbidopa-levodopa, but the drug's effect gradually wears off in: *(207)*
    1. 12 to 24 months.
    2. 3 to 5 years.
    3. 1 to 2 years.
    4. 6 to 8 months.

20. When patients start on monoamine oxidase type B inhibitor therapy in conjunction with carbidopa-levodopa (Sinemet), the dosages of Sinemet can be titrated downward starting at: *(206)*
    1. month 4 or 5 of therapy.
    2. month 2 or 3 of therapy.
    3. week 2 or 3 of therapy.
    4. day 2 or 3 of therapy.

21. When the drugs used for Parkinson's disease start to become ineffective, it is known as: *(205)*
    1. hypermobility.
    2. common adverse effect.
    3. neuroprotective.
    4. on-off phenomenon.

Cite the action of carbidopa, levodopa, and apomorphine on the neurotransmitters involved in Parkinson's disease.

22. The major action of the drug carbidopa-levodopa (Sinemet) is to: *(207)*
    1. reduce dopamine production.
    2. reduce metabolism of levodopa.
    3. increase the metabolism of levodopa.
    4. absorb more levodopa.

23. The drug carbidopa-levodopa (Sinemet) must be given in combination because: *(207)*
    1. levodopa is used to reduce the dose of carbidopa required.
    2. levodopa has no effect when used alone.
    3. carbidopa has no effect when used alone.
    4. carbidopa is used to increase the dose of levodopa required.

24. Which are nursing considerations for patients on apomorphine (Apokyn) therapy? *(Select all that apply.) (210)*
    1. Administer prochlorperazine (Compazine) for nausea associated with apomorphine therapy.
    2. Assess patients on apomorphine therapy for orthostatic hypotension.
    3. Calculate apomorphine dose based on milligrams.
    4. Do not administer apomorphine intravenously.
    5. Assess patients receiving apomorphine therapy for sudden sleep attacks.

Explain the action of entacapone and of the monoamine oxidase inhibitors (selegiline and rasagiline) as it relates to the treatment of Parkinson's disease.

25. The major action of the drug entacapone (Comtan), which is a COMT inhibitor, is to: *(214)*
    1. increase the absorption of dopamine.
    2. slow the progression of deterioration of dopaminergic nerve cells.
    3. increase the adverse dopaminergic effects of levodopa.
    4. reduce the destruction of dopamine in the peripheral tissues.

26. Active metabolites of selegiline, when swallowed, are amphetamines that cause cardiovascular and psychiatric adverse effects. To avoid this effect, the drug is administered as (a)n: *(206)*
    1. rectal suppository.
    2. subcutaneous injection.
    3. orally disintegrating tablet.
    4. intradermal injection.
27. The major action of the drug rasagiline is considered neuroprotective, which: *(205)*
    1. increases the absorption of dopamine.
    2. slows the rate of deterioration of the dopamine neurons.
    3. reduces the destruction of dopamine in the peripheral tissues.
    4. slows the rate of symptoms in the later stages of Parkinson's disease.

Describe the symptoms that can be attributed to the cholinergic activity of pharmacologic agents.

28. The main reason anticholinergic agents are prescribed for patients with parkinsonism is to: *(215)*
    1. decrease the absorption of acetylcholine.
    2. increase the absorption of dopamine.
    3. reduce hyperstimulation caused by the excess amount of acetylcholine.
    4. prevent the adverse effect of orthostatic hypotension.
29. Anticholinergic agents produce which effects? *(Select all that apply.) (216)*
    1. Dry mouth
    2. Diarrhea
    3. Runny nose
    4. Dry nose
    5. Constipation

30. The symptoms that are targeted for treatment when anticholinergic agents are used include: *(Select all that apply.) (215)*
    1. postural abnormalities.
    2. drooling.
    3. rigidity.
    4. bradykinesia.
    5. tremors.

Cite the specific symptoms that should show improvement when anticholinergic agents are administered to a patient with Parkinson's disease.

31. After being treated for Parkinson's disease, patients will demonstrate improvement in their symptoms by: *(Select all that apply.) (215)*
    1. improved gait.
    2. decreased depression.
    3. improved speech.
    4. increased drooling.
    5. decreased tremors.
32. Long-term use of levodopa can cause abnormal movements such as: *(Select all that apply.) (208)*
    1. chewing motions.
    2. rocking.
    3. head and neck bobbing.
    4. facial grimacing.
    5. increased swallowing.
33. The therapeutic outcomes desired when an anticholinergic agent is prescribed for a Parkinson's patient include: *(Select all that apply.) (215)*
    1. reduced drooling.
    2. increased sweating.
    3. increased depression.
    4. reduced tremors.
    5. head and neck bobbing.

Drugs Used for Anxiety Disorders

chapter

15

Answer Key: Textbook page references are provided as a guide for answering these questions. A complete answer key is provided to your instructor.

MATCHING

Match the definition on the right with the term on the left.

Term		Definition
1.	_____ anxiety	a. an abrupt surge of intense fear or intense discomfort
2.	_____ panic	b. excessive and unrealistic worry about two or more life circumstances
3.	_____ phobias	c. recurrent thoughts or actions that cause significant distress interfere with normal functioning
4.	_____ obsessive-compulsive	d. irrational fears of specific objects, activities, or situations

REVIEW QUESTIONS

Scenario: A 58-year-old patient was admitted for further evaluation of bizarre behavior manifested as loud, rapid talking; pacing; and wringing of the hands. Relatives have attempted to calm the patient with no effect, and they brought the patient to urgent care for consultation.

Compare and contrast the differences between generalized anxiety disorder, panic disorder, phobias, and obsessive-compulsive disorder.

5. When patients have irrational fears of a specific object, activity, or situation, and even recognize the fear as exaggerated or unrealistic, this is termed: *(219)*
   1. phobia.
   2. panic disorder.
   3. obsessive-compulsive disorder.
   4. allergic response.
6. Anxiety is a component of many medical illnesses involving which systems? *(Select all that apply.) (218)*
   1. Cardiovascular
   2. Pulmonary
   3. Digestive
   4. Endocrine
   5. Sensory
7. When patients have unwanted thoughts, ideas, images, or an urge that the patient recognizes as time-consuming and senseless but repeatedly intrudes into the consciousness despite attempts to ignore, prevent, or counteract it, the patient is said to be experiencing: *(219)*
   1. phobia.
   2. panic disorder.
   3. obsessive-compulsive disorder.
   4. an allergic response.

Describe the essential components included in a baseline assessment of a patient's mental status.

8. In the scenario, the nurse will regularly assess the patient for which symptoms to determine if acute hospitalization is indicated? *(220-221)*
   1. Patient appears to be at risk for harming him- or herself or others.
   2. Patient has a clean and neat appearance, and the ability to perform self-care.
   3. Patient demonstrates a stooped or slumped posture, and is oriented to date, time, place, and person.
   4. Patient is complaining of nausea and refuses breakfast.
9. It is important for the nurse to identify events that trigger anxiety such as: *(Select all that apply.) (219)*
   1. social or performance situation.
   2. spiders, snakes, and mice.
   3. being in a crowded place.
   4. genetic component.
   5. nonstimulating environment.
10. The nurse is taking care of the patient in the scenario and performs a baseline mental status assessment, which will include asking the patient to describe his or her normal patterns of: *(Select all that apply.) (220-221)*
    1. family interactions.

2. sleep.
3. psychomotor functions.
4. obsessions or compulsions.
5. dietary history.

Cite the drug therapy used to treat anxiety disorders listed in objective 1.

11. The drug classes used to treat patients with anxiety disorders include: (*Select all that apply.*) **(219)**
    1. selective serotonin reuptake inhibitors (SSRIs).
    2. azaspirones.
    3. calcium channel blockers.
    4. benzodiazepines.
    5. monoamine oxidase type B inhibitors.

12. Hydroxyzine therapy is used for patients who suffer from conditions characterized by anxiety, tension, and agitation, because it has which effect? **(225)**
    1. Antihistaminic
    2. Antiemetic
    3. Antianxiety
    4. Antispasmodic

13. The nursing implications for buspirone therapy include watching for adverse effects of the drug such as: (*Select all that apply.*) **(224)**
    1. dizziness and insomnia.
    2. orthostatic hypotension.
    3. sedation and lethargy.
    4. nervousness and drowsiness.
    5. restless leg syndrome.

14. The benzodiazepine drug monograph lists hepatotoxicity as a serious adverse effect. Which laboratory tests are performed to assess this? **(224)**
    1. Bilirubin, alkaline phosphatase, gamma-glutamyltransferase (GGT), and prothrombin time
    2. Albumin, ferritin, and prothrombin time
    3. Aspartate aminotransferase (AST), GGT, and ferritin
    4. Creatinine, creatinine clearance, and albumin

Identify adverse effects that may result from drug therapy used to treat anxiety.

15. When determining if drug therapy is effective for patients taking meprobamate as an antianxiety agent, the nurse will note which characteristics of the patient's behavior? (*Select all that apply.*) **(226)**
    1. Coping has improved.
    2. Physical signs of anxiety are reduced.
    3. Slurred speech and dizziness occur.
    4. Physical signs of anxiety such as pacing have increased.
    5. The patient is able to work around machinery.

16. Those patients who experience anxiety with other conditions are treated with benzodiazepine therapy because they: **(223)**
    1. generally will not tolerate fluoxetine or any other SSRI.

2. will respond most readily with a reduction in anxiety.
3. respond to behavior therapy better than drugs.
4. will not have any recurrence of symptoms after treatment.

17. Nurses need to teach patients taking hydroxyzine therapy for anxiety to report which symptoms that should be monitored? **(226)**
    1. Morning hangover
    2. Reduction in anxiety
    3. Excessive sedation
    4. Dry mouth

18. What information does the nurse include during patient teaching for antianxiety therapy? **(223)**
    1. "You may take this medication while operating machinery."
    2. "When discontinuing the medication, there is no need to reduce the dose gradually."
    3. "Notify your healthcare provider if hangover symptoms persist, because the dose may need to be reduced or the medication changed."
    4. "Therapeutic effects of the drug take 4 to 6 weeks to occur."

19. Which drugs may increase the toxic effects of benzodiazepines? (*Select all that apply.*) **(224)**
    1. Antihistamines
    2. Alcohol
    3. Analgesics
    4. Beta blockers
    5. Beta-adrenergic agonists

Discuss psychological and physiologic drug dependence.

20. When a patient is withdrawn from long-term use of benzodiazepines, the nurse assesses for which signs/symptoms? (*Select all that apply.*) **(223)**
    1. Restlessness
    2. Worsening of anxiety
    3. Tremors
    4. Decreased heart rate
    5. Auditory hypersensitivity

21. The nurse is assessing a patient before administering buspirone (BuSpar). Which finding would the nurse call the prescriber about to determine the appropriateness of the drug? **(224)**
    1. Slurred speech
    2. Insomnia
    3. Nervousness
    4. Dizziness

22. Psychological and physiologic dependence may occur in patients taking meprobamate. Symptoms of chronic use and abuse of high doses include: (*Select all that apply.*) **(226)**
    1. ataxia.
    2. confusion.
    3. slurred speech.
    4. dizziness.
    5. hallucinations.

Drugs Used for Depressive and Bipolar Disorders

chapter
16

Answer Key: Textbook page references are provided as a guide for answering these questions. A complete answer key is provided to your instructor.

MATCHING

Match the drug classification on the right with the drug name on the left. Classifications may be used more than once.

	Drug Name		**Drug Classification**
1. _____	citalopram (Celexa)	a.	MAOI
2. _____	venlafaxine (Effexor)	b.	TCA
3. _____	isocarboxazid (Marplan)	c.	SSRI
4. _____	imipramine (Tofranil PM)	d.	SNRI
5. _____	selegiline (Emsam)		
6. _____	duloxetine (Cymbalta)		
7. _____	clomipramine (Anafranil)		
8. _____	escitalopram (Lexapro)		

REVIEW QUESTIONS

Scenario: A 78-year-old patient came into the clinic complaining of insomnia and lack of motivation to do daily activities, which has been increasing in occurrence for the last several months.

Describe the essential components of the baseline assessment of a patient with depression or bipolar disorder.

9. Characteristic symptoms found in a person experiencing depression include: *(Select all that apply.)* **(229)**
   1. persistent lack of motivation.
   2. sadness.
   3. inability to concentrate.
   4. slowed thinking.
   5. sudden personality change.
10. The patient in the scenario is likely suffering from: **(229)**
    1. bipolar disorder.
    2. labile mood.
    3. depression.
    4. mania.
11. The nurse is assessing a patient who is being started on imipramine (Tofranil) and is reviewing the basic components of the assessment for mood disorders,

which include asking the patient about: *(Select all that apply.)* **(232-233)**
   1. job expectations.
   2. interpersonal relationships.
   3. hygiene habits.
   4. history of mood disorders.
   5. thoughts of death.
12. Bipolar disorder is characterized by: **(229-230)**
   1. pacing, hand-wringing, and outbursts of shouting.
   2. episodes of mania and depression separated by intervals without mood disturbances.
   3. slowed thinking, confusion, and poor memory.
   4. alternating episodes of mania and depression.
13. Symptoms of acute mania occurring during the manic phase of bipolar disorder may include: *(Select all that apply.)* **(230)**
   1. increased need for sleep.
   2. gradual onset of symptoms that takes several weeks.
   3. heightened mood.
   4. paranoia.
   5. increased energy.
14. Patients experiencing the manic phase of bipolar disorder generally: **(230)**
   1. develop a stable mood during this phase.

2. recognize the symptoms of illness in themselves.
3. do not recognize the symptoms of illness in themselves.
4. will not develop psychotic symptoms.

Identify the premedication assessments that are necessary before the administration of MAOIs, SNRIs, TCAs, and antimanic agents.

15. When patients experience the physiologic manifestations of depression such as sleep disturbance, change in appetite, loss of energy, fatigue, or palpitations, they can expect to have relief from these symptoms within the: *(232)*
    1. first week of starting therapy.
    2. second week of starting therapy.
    3. third week of starting therapy.
    4. fourth week of starting therapy.
16. The adverse effects that tend to develop early in therapy for patients with depression result in: *(234)*
    1. decreased thought processes.
    2. noncompliance.
    3. delusions of grandeur.
    4. personality change.
17. The treatment of mood disorders requires nonpharmacologic and pharmacologic therapy, and may include: *(Select all that apply.) (230-231)*
    1. electroconvulsive therapy.
    2. psychodynamic therapy.
    3. cognitive-behavioral therapy.
    4. personality inventory.
    5. pharmacologic treatment.
18. The premedication assessment that nurses perform for TCAs includes: *(Select all that apply.) (241-242)*
    1. noting constituency of the patient's stools, to watch for constipation.
    2. taking the patient's blood pressure and report hypotension.
    3. obtaining the patient's height and weight.
    4. checking for a history of seizures.
    5. determining if there is any history of dysrhythmias.
19. The medication assessment that nurses perform for antimanic agents includes: *(Select all that apply.) (250)*
    1. monitoring lithium levels once or twice weekly during the start of therapy.
    2. obtaining laboratory tests such as electrolytes, blood glucose, and blood urea nitrogen (BUN).
    3. obtaining baseline blood pressures supine, sitting, and standing.
    4. weighing the patient weekly.
    5. administering the antimanic agent on an empty stomach.

Compare the mechanism of action of selective serotonin reuptake inhibitors (SSRIs) with that of other antidepressant agents.

20. SSRIs act by: *(239)*

1. an unknown exact mechanism of action.
2. blocking the destruction of serotonin.
3. inhibiting the reuptake of serotonin.
4. inhibiting the degradation of serotonin.

21. SSRIs are the most widely used class of antidepressants because they have been shown to be effective and: *(239)*
    1. can be safely administered to children.
    2. only have anticholinergic adverse effects.
    3. are less costly.
    4. do not have the adverse effects of other antidepressants.
22. SSRIs are being studied to identify if these agents can successfully be used to treat other disorders such as: *(Select all that apply.) (239)*
    1. diabetic retinopathy.
    2. anorexia nervosa.
    3. autism.
    4. panic disorders.
    5. menopausal symptoms.
23. Which SSRI is approved for treatment of depression in children and adolescents? *(239)*
    1. Sertraline (Zoloft)
    2. Fluoxetine (Prozac)
    3. Paroxetine (Paxil)
    4. Fluvoxamine (Luvox)
24. SSRIs have an advantage over tricyclic antidepressants because they do not: *(239)*
    1. require suicidal precautions be in place.
    2. take 2 to 4 weeks of therapy to obtain the therapeutic effect.
    3. cause anticholinergic and cardiovascular adverse effects compared to tricyclic antidepressants.
    4. cause insomnia or restlessness.

Cite the common adverse effects that may develop for patients who are taking monoamine oxidase inhibitors (MAOIs).

25. When patients are taking MAOIs, the nurse needs to instruct patients on: *(Select all that apply.) (238)*
    1. how to limit tyramine-containing foods in their diet.
    2. the importance of not discontinuing the drug abruptly.
    3. taking the divided dose no later than 8 PM.
    4. dividing the dose to prevent drug-induced insomnia.
    5. the drugs that are known to cause drug interactions.
26. When patients are taking the MAOI selegiline (Emsam), the nurse needs to assess for: *(238)*
    1. dizziness and weakness.
    2. therapeutic serum levels.
    3. decreased sedation.
    4. diarrhea.
27. The nurse was instructing a diabetic patient who was starting on the MAOI isocarboxazid (Marplan)

regarding precautions to use, and realized further education was needed after the patient stated: *(237)*
1. "Since I have to take insulin, I will need to adjust my doses while I take this drug."
2. "As I understand it, I can stop taking my insulin since this drug will cause hypoglycemia."
3. "I get it; I need to carefully monitor my blood sugar while I am on this drug."
4. "I will need to carefully determine what foods I can eat while on this drug."

Cite the common adverse effects that may develop for patients who are taking serotonin-norepinephrine reuptake inhibitors (SNRIs).

28. Nursing implications for patients taking SNRI therapy include: *(Select all that apply.)* *(240-241)*
    1. making certain that patients taper their dosage over several days when discontinuing the drug.
    2. tapering venlafaxine over 2 weeks if taken for longer than 6 weeks when discontinuing the drug.
    3. recognizing improvement may take up to 6 weeks.
    4. understanding that depression will be alleviated entirely with therapy.
    5. knowing suicide precautions should be maintained during first several weeks of therapy.

29. What do nurses need to assess for in patients prior to starting therapy with the SNRI duloxetine (Cymbalta)? *(Select all that apply.)* *(240)*
    1. GI symptoms
    2. Glaucoma
    3. Insomnia
    4. Hypertension
    5. Thyroid disorders

30. Nurses need to explain to patients that they cannot work with machinery or operate a motor vehicle if they develop which adverse effect? *(241)*
    1. Restlessness, anxiety, or agitation
    2. Insomnia
    3. Dizziness or drowsiness
    4. Nausea or anorexia

Cite the common adverse effects that may develop for patients who are taking tricyclic antidepressants (TCAs).

31. When patients are taking TCAs for depression, the most important baseline parameter the nurse needs to assess is: *(241)*
    1. weight.
    2. blood pressure in supine and sitting positions.

3. temperature.
4. pulse.

32. Primary outcomes expected from TCAs include elevated mood and reduction of symptoms of depression, and TCAs can also be used for the treatment of: *(Select all that apply.)* *(241)*
    1. chronic pain.
    2. eating disorders.
    3. obstructive sleep apnea.
    4. benign prostatic hyperplasia.
    5. seizures.

33. Selected TCAs are also used to treat other disorders such as: *(Select all that apply.)* *(241)*
    1. phantom limb pain.
    2. arthritic pain.
    3. premenstrual symptoms.
    4. cancer pain.
    5. menopause symptoms.

Cite the common adverse effects that may develop for patients who are taking lithium.

34. The drug most commonly used to treat the manic phase of bipolar disorder is: *(249)*
    1. citalopram (Celexa).
    2. lithium carbonate (Eskalith).
    3. duloxetine (Cymbalta).
    4. venlafaxine (Effexor).

35. When the antimanic agent lithium is used for patients with bipolar disorder, the nurse educates the patient and family on which ways to prevent toxicity? *(Select all that apply.)* *(250)*
    1. "You will need to monitor your lithium levels once or twice weekly during the start of this therapy."
    2. "Lithium needs to be taken with food or milk."
    3. "You will need to maintain a normal dietary intake of sodium with adequate water."
    4. "The full therapeutic effect of this drug often requires 21 to 30 days."
    5. "You need to report immediately any persistent vomiting and diarrhea, as these are signs of toxicity."

36. The nurse needs to assess for early signs of lithium toxicity, which include: *(Select all that apply.)* *(250)*
    1. increased appetite.
    2. muscle twitching and tremors.
    3. nausea and vomiting.
    4. lethargy.
    5. speech difficulties.

Drugs Used for Psychoses

chapter
17

Answer Key: Textbook page references are provided as a guide for answering these questions. A complete answer key is provided to your instructor.

MATCHING
Match the term on the right with the definition on the left.

Definition

1. _____ spasmodic movements of muscle groups

2. _____ a syndrome of persistent and involuntary hyperkinetic abnormal movements

3. _____ tremors, muscle rigidity, mask-like expressions, shuffling gait, and loss or weakness of motor function

4. _____ a syndrome of anxiety and restlessness, and associated pacing, rocking, and an inability to sit or stand in one place for extended periods

Term

a. pseudoparkinsonian symptoms
b. akathisia
c. tardive dyskinesia
d. dystonia

REVIEW QUESTIONS

Scenario: A 45-year-old male patient was admitted to the inpatient psychiatric unit for further evaluation and treatment after he was found by his family to be babbling incoherently and rapidly pacing in his apartment. He has a history of schizoid affective disorder and had not taken his medications lately.

Identify the signs and symptoms of psychotic behavior.

5. The patient is said to be suffering from psychosis when which of these symptoms are present? *(Select all that apply.)* **(253)**
   1. Hallucinations
   2. Orthostatic hypotension
   3. Insomnia
   4. Delusions
   5. Disorganized thinking

6. A patient in the emergency department tells the nurse that he is the creator of the universe. What does the nurse suspect that this patient is experiencing? **(253)**
   1. Disorganized thinking
   2. Change of affect
   3. Hallucinations
   4. Delusions

7. Target symptoms are critical monitoring parameters used to assess changes in the patient's status and his or her response to medications. Examples of target symptoms include: *(Select all that apply.)* **(254)**
   1. weight gain.
   2. degree of suspiciousness.
   3. substance abuse.
   4. type of agitation.
   5. loose associations.

Describe the major indications for the use of antipsychotic agents.

8. Underlying disorders which may cause psychosis may not necessitate the use of antipsychotic agents, but rather the treatment of the disorder such as: *(Select all that apply.)* **(253)**
   1. infections.
   2. endocrine disorders.
   3. schizophrenia.
   4. bipolar disorders.
   5. metabolic disturbances.

9. Psychotic symptoms common with mood disorders that necessitate the patient being started on an antipsychotic agent include: *(Select all that apply.)* **(253)**
   1. schizophrenia.
   2. bipolar disorder.
   3. anorexia.

4. major depression.
5. obsessive-compulsive disorder.

10. The nurse includes in teaching the patient in the scenario that taking antipsychotic agents may cause dystonic reactions, which may: *(258)*
    1. occur most often in the first 72 hours of therapy.
    2. occur most often in females.
    3. not be responsive to treatment.
    4. usually last for 1 week.

Discuss the antipsychotic medications that are used for the treatment of psychoses.

11. First-generation antipsychotic agents are the phenothiazines, which are thought to: *(262-263)*
    1. block serotonin reuptake inhibitors.
    2. block the serotonin receptors.
    3. block dopamine in the CNS.
    4. release serotonin at the receptor sites.

12. The second-generation or atypical antipsychotic agents are thought to: *(263)*
    1. block serotonin reuptake inhibitors.
    2. block the dopamine and serotonin receptors.
    3. block dopamine in the CNS.
    4. release serotonin at the receptor sites.

13. Atypical antipsychotic agents are most commonly used because they tend to be more effective in relieving negative symptoms. These agents include: *(Select all that apply.)* *(263)*
    1. haloperidol (Haldol).
    2. risperidone (Risperdal).
    3. quetiapine (Seroquel).

4. aripiprazole (Abilify).
5. ziprasidone (Geodon).

Identify the common adverse effects that are observed with the use of antipsychotic medications.

14. The nurse will discuss with the patient in the scenario who is taking an antipsychotic drug that he may experience which adverse effects? *(Select all that apply.)* *(263-264)*
    1. Tardive dyskinesia
    2. Weight loss
    3. Hypoglycemia
    4. Orthostatic hypotension
    5. Seizures

15. Patients taking antipsychotic medications may experience which adverse effects as a result of the anticholinergic effects produced by these agents? *(Select all that apply.)* *(263)*
    1. Diarrhea
    2. Chronic fatigue
    3. Dry mouth
    4. Blurred vision
    5. Urinary retention

16. A patient has been started on the atypical antipsychotic clozapine (Clozaril) for bipolar disorder. For the first 6 months of therapy, which lab result is most important for the nurse to monitor? *(263)*
    1. Red blood cell counts
    2. White blood cell counts
    3. Blood glucose
    4. Thyroid-stimulating hormone

Drugs Used for Seizure Disorders

Answer Key: Textbook page references are provided as a guide for answering these questions. A complete answer key is provided to your instructor.

MATCHING
Match the drug classification on the right with the drug name on the left. Classifications may be used more than once.

Drug Name

1. _____ carbamazepine (Tegretol)
2. _____ clonazepam (Tranxene)
3. _____ ethosuximide (Zarontin)
4. _____ gabapentin (Neurontin)
5. _____ lamotrigine (Lamictal)
6. _____ levetiracetam (Keppra)
7. _____ phenytoin (Dilantin)
8. _____ topiramate (Topamax)
9. _____ zonisamide (Zonegran)

Drug Classification

a. benzodiazepines
b. hydantoins
c. succinimides
d. phenyltriazine
e. pyrrolidine
f. sulfonamide
g. miscellaneous anticonvulsants

REVIEW QUESTIONS

Scenario: A 32-year-old female was admitted to the hospital following an episode of a generalized seizure witnessed by her husband.

Identify the different types of seizure disorders.

10. During which types of seizures is it not uncommon for patients to lose their balance and fall with no loss of consciousness? *(267)*
    1. Tonic-clonic and myoclonic
    2. Myoclonic and atonic
    3. Atonic and tonic-clonic
    4. Absence and myoclonic
11. When monitoring a patient during a seizure, the nurse knows that atonic or akinetic seizures manifest as: *(267)*
    1. bilateral jerks alternating with relaxation of the extremities.
    2. intense muscular contractions.
    3. a sudden loss of muscle tone, occurring in short attacks.
    4. lightning-like repetitive contractions of the muscles of the face.

12. Which type of seizure is considered a medical emergency and prompt treatment is necessary to prevent nerve damage and death? *(267)*
    1. Myoclonic seizures
    2. Tonic-clonic seizures
    3. Absence seizures
    4. Status epilepticus
13. Seizures are divided into which classifications? *(266)*
    1. Generalized seizures and partial seizures
    2. Grand mal seizures and petit mal seizures
    3. Generalized convulsive seizures and generalized nonconvulsive seizures
    4. Full seizures and partial seizures

Identify nursing interventions during the management of seizure activity.

14. The nurse needs to educate the patient in the scenario on what to expect from the seizure medications, as well as common adverse effects that may occur, which include: *(Select all that apply.)* *(274)*
    1. nausea and vomiting.
    2. blood dyscrasias.
    3. orthostatic hypotension.
    4. dizziness.
    5. drowsiness.

15. Which action does the nurse take when working with a patient experiencing a seizure? *(269)*
    1. Restrains the patient
    2. Places a tongue blade in the patient's mouth
    3. Once the patient enters into the recovery phase, turns him or her slightly onto the side to allow secretions to drain from the mouth
    4. Medicates the patient immediately
16. The nurse is discussing the diagnosis of epilepsy to parents of a 5-year-old child who had been recently diagnosed with tonic-clonic seizures. Which statement by the parents indicates that the nurse needs to educate further? *(267)*
    1. "Seizures are grouped into two types, generalized and partial."
    2. "*Epilepsy* is the general term meaning that the seizures are chronic."
    3. "The tonic-clonic seizures that were diagnosed have a recovery stage."
    4. "These seizures will be outgrown later in life."
17. Nurses need to document what is happening to a patient during a seizure and include which information regarding the seizure? *(Select all that apply.)* *(269-270)*
    1. Progression of symptoms
    2. Onset or possible causal factor
    3. Duration
    4. State of consciousness
    5. Which hemisphere of the brain is being affected
18. The nurse is teaching the patient in the scenario about the use of phenytoin (Dilantin) for seizure control. What does the nurse tell the patient about taking oral contraceptives with this medication? *(274)*
    1. "You will not be able to become pregnant because of the phenytoin therapy."
    2. "Dilantin therapy should be stopped if you experience spotting or bleeding."
    3. "An alternative form of birth control should be used when taking phenytoin with oral contraceptives."
    4. "There are no contraindications for using these two drugs together."

Cite the desired therapeutic outcomes from antiepileptic agents used for seizure disorders.

19. When administering antiepileptic agents to patients, the nurse knows that the therapeutic outcomes include: *(Select all that apply.)* *(267)*
    1. reduced frequency of seizures.
    2. reduced injury from seizure activity.
    3. minimal adverse effects from therapy.
    4. reduced tension and stress.
    5. alleviating any seizure activity.
20. The drug of choice for controlling the seizure activity of patient in the scenario is: *(268)*
    1. lorazepam (Ativan).
    2. gabapentin (Neurontin).
    3. pregabalin (Lyrica).
    4. topiramate (Topamax).

21. Alternative(s) to the drug of choice for the patient in the scenario if the first one did not work to control the seizures would include: *(Select all that apply.)* *(268)*
    1. levetiracetam (Keppra).
    2. gabapentin (Neurontin).
    3. phenytoin (Dilantin).
    4. topiramate (Topamax).
    5. lamotrigine (Lamictal).

Identify the drug classes used to treat seizure disorders.

22. Benzodiazepines are used for the treatment of seizures because they are thought to: *(271)*
    1. enhance the effects of gamma-aminobutyric acid (GABA).
    2. cause the destruction of GABA.
    3. prevent the breakdown of dopamine.
    4. prevent reuptake of GABA.
23. Succinimides are drugs that are used to decrease the frequency of seizures by which mechanism of action? *(275)*
    1. Blocking the reuptake of norepinephrine
    2. Preventing the breakdown of dopamine
    3. Enhancing the effects of GABA
    4. Reducing the current in the T-type calcium channels
24. The miscellaneous antiepileptic agent carbamazepine (Tegretol) works by: *(275)*
    1. decreasing the effectiveness of GABA.
    2. blocking the reuptake of norepinephrine.
    3. increasing the effectiveness of GABA.
    4. increasing the rate of dopamine being released.
25. The newer anticonvulsant lamotrigine, unrelated to other antiepileptic medications, is thought to act by blocking voltage-sensitive sodium and calcium channels, and is part of which class of drugs? *(278)*
    1. Sulfonamides
    2. Phenyltriazine
    3. Succinimides
    4. Pyrrolidine

Describe the neurologic assessment performed on patients taking antiepileptic agents to monitor for common and serious adverse effects.

26. Patients who are diabetic and taking hydantoins need to be educated on the risk of: *(273)*
    1. developing oral thrush.
    2. decreased effectiveness of hydantoin.
    3. hyperglycemia with hydantoin therapy.
    4. increased frequency of hypoglycemia.
27. When patients are on antacids and hydantoins, they should be told that the antacid will: *(274)*
    1. increase the level of hydantoin in the blood.
    2. decrease the therapeutic effects of the hydantoin.
    3. have an increased effectiveness.
    4. have a decreased effectiveness.

28. The nurse assessing the patient in the scenario who is starting on topiramate (Topamax) knows to monitor for common adverse effects such as: *(Select all that apply.)* **(285)**
    1. sedation.
    2. drowsiness.
    3. increased sweating.
    4. dizziness.
    5. constipation.

Drugs Used for Pain Management

Answer Key: Textbook page references are provided as a guide for answering these questions. A complete answer key is provided to your instructor.

MATCHING

Match the definition on the right with the term on the left.

	Term		Definition
1.	_____ pain experience	a.	the point at which an individual first acknowledges or interprets a sensation of pain
2.	_____ pain perception	b.	an individual's awareness of the feeling or sensation of pain
3.	_____ pain threshold	c.	the individual's ability to endure pain
4.	_____ pain tolerance	d.	an unpleasant sensation that is highly subjective and influenced by sensory, emotional, and cultural factors

REVIEW QUESTIONS

Scenario: A patient recovering from a recent fall that resulted in broken vertebrae and the need for a turtle shell for back support was talking with a nurse about pain control.

Describe the pain assessment used for patients receiving opiate agonists.

5. The nurse in the scenario is discussing various pain management options with the patient and realizes more education is needed when the patient states: *(297)*
   1. "I will keep taking the narcotic every 4 hours until I run out."
   2. "I need to taper the amount of narcotic I am taking and supplement Tylenol or Advil."
   3. "I know I need to switch from taking so much narcotic because I am getting constipated."
   4. "I will start to take more Tylenol or Advil during the day and more narcotic at night so I can sleep."

6. For patients taking opiate agonists, the nurse needs to monitor the patient for signs of: *(Select all that apply.) (303)*
   1. respiratory depression.
   2. urinary retention.
   3. diarrhea.
   4. confusion or disorientation.
   5. hyperglycemia.

7. When determining if the patient has adequate relief from pain, the nurse needs to assess which compo-

nents of the pain assessment? *(Select all that apply.)* *(296)*
   1. The onset, or what activates pain
   2. The quality of pain; whether it is described as stabbing, dull, burning, etc.
   3. The duration, or how long the pain persists
   4. How the patient rates the pain on a pain scale
   5. The last time no pain was felt

Differentiate among the properties of opiate agonists, opiate partial agonists, and opiate antagonists.

8. The nurse understands that opiate agonists interact with receptors to stimulate a response of pain relief, whereas partial agonists may: *(304)*
   1. block any response.
   2. stimulate a response, but may inhibit other responses.
   3. induce a stupor or sleep.
   4. induce withdrawal symptoms if any opiate agonist has been given.

9. The mechanism of action for opiate antagonists is to: *(306)*
   1. block the effects of any euphoric high.
   2. stimulate a response, but may inhibit other responses.
   3. stimulate a response of pain relief.
   4. reverse the depressant effects of any opiate agonist.

10. The nurse knows that which is true about the use of the transdermal opioid analgesic fentanyl (Duragesic)? *(301)*

1. Fentanyl is only used for acute pain.
2. Approximately 2 hours are required for the initial patch of medication to reach a steady blood level.
3. Fentanyl patches provide relief for up to 72 hours.
4. No other analgesics may be used concurrently with fentanyl.

Cite the common adverse effects of opiate agonists.

11. The patient in the scenario is receiving opiate agonists for pain control. Which adverse effect does the nurse report to the healthcare provider? *(Select all that apply.)* *(303)*
    1. Lightheadedness
    2. Respiratory rate of 7
    3. Dry mouth
    4. Urinary retention
    5. Daily bowel movements
12. Which common adverse effect can usually be treated by diet and stool softeners? *(303)*
    1. Respiratory depression
    2. Urinary retention
    3. Constipation
    4. Orthostatic hypotension
13. Patients who report lightheadedness and dizziness after the first dose of hydromorphone (Dilaudid) should be instructed by the nurse to: *(303)*
    1. increase the amount of whole-grain products in their diet.
    2. remain lying down.
    3. report this effect to the healthcare provider for further evaluation.
    4. sit up quickly and stand after 30 seconds of sitting to relieve symptoms.
14. If an opiate partial agonist (nalbuphine) is administered to a patient who is addicted to opiate agonists (oxycodone), what must the nurse assess for? *(304)*
    1. Withdrawal symptoms
    2. Constipation
    3. Hypotension
    4. Elevated WBCs
15. What drugs are antidotes for opiate agonists and opiate partial agonists? *(304)*
    1. Naloxone (Evzio) and pentazocine (Talwin)
    2. Naltrexone (ReVia) and nalbuphine (Nubain)
    3. Naloxone (Evzio) and naltrexone (ReVia)
    4. Naltrexone (ReVia) and butorphanol (Stadol)
16. When are opiate partial agonists effective in relieving pain? *(304)*
    1. In people who have recently taken opiate agonists
    2. After opiate agonists are no longer effective
    3. For patients after surgery in conjunction with opiate agonists
    4. In cases without prior administration of opiate agonists

Describe the three pharmacologic effects of salicylates.

17. Salicylates are known to have which pharmacologic properties? *(309)*
    1. Antiepileptic, antiplatelet, and antiinflammatory
    2. Analgesic, antiplatelet, and antacid
    3. Analgesic, antipyretic, and antiinflammatory
    4. Antiinflammatory, antipyretic, and antacid
18. Salicylates are used for which conditions? *(Select all that apply.)* *(309)*
    1. Relief of inflammation from rheumatoid arthritis
    2. Reduce fever from infections
    3. Prevent the symptoms of withdrawal from opiates
    4. Reduce the risk of recurrent TIA or stroke
    5. Reduce the risk of myocardial infarction
19. Salicylates work by inhibiting prostaglandins, which cause: *(Select all that apply.)* *(309)*
    1. platelets to aggregate.
    2. sensitization of the pain receptors that cause pain.
    3. elevation of body temperature.
    4. mental sluggishness and sedation.
    5. signs and symptoms of inflammation.

List the common and serious adverse effects and drug interactions associated with salicylates.

20. A patient has been taking an oral hypoglycemic agent and is being started on salicylate therapy for pain management. What does the nurse anticipate will happen when these two types of drugs are taken together? *(309)*
    1. The patient will need to switch to subcutaneous insulin therapy for the duration of the salicylate therapy.
    2. The oral hypoglycemic agent will potentiate the effect of the salicylate and increase the chance of salicylate toxicity.
    3. The dose of the oral hypoglycemic agent will be doubled while the patient is on salicylate therapy.
    4. Salicylates may enhance the hypoglycemic effects of oral hypoglycemic agents; therefore, the dose may need to be reduced.
21. Salicylates should not be used in children because of the associated risk of: *(309)*
    1. overdose.
    2. Reye's syndrome.
    3. toxic response.
    4. respiratory depression.
22. Salicylates should not be given when patients have which conditions? *(Select all that apply.)* *(310)*
    1. Gastric ulcers
    2. Previous myocardial infarctions
    3. Coagulation disorders
    4. Glaucoma
    5. Liver disease

23. When comparing the therapeutic effects of NSAIDs to acetaminophen (Tylenol), the nurse knows that both are very good antipyretic and analgesic agents; however: *(308)*
    1. acetaminophen has antiplatelet effects.
    2. NSAIDs have antiplatelet effects.
    3. acetaminophen has no antiinflammatory effect.
    4. NSAIDs are effective when used with opiate agonists.
24. The primary therapeutic outcomes expected from acetaminophen (Tylenol) are: *(308)*
    1. reduced inflammation and pain.
    2. reduced pain and fever.
    3. relief from pain and heartburn.
    4. improved circulation and nasal congestion.
25. The three commonly used NSAIDs are: *(314)*
    1. ibuprofen (Advil), indomethacin (Indocin), ketorolac (Toradol).
    2. meloxicam (Mobic), naproxen (Aleve), diflunisal (Dolobid).
    3. celecoxib (Celebrex), oxaprozin (Daypro), butorphanol (Stadol).
    4. sulindac (Clinoril), celecoxib (Celebrex), pentazocine (Talwin).
26. The nurse is explaining to the patient in the scenario that the active ingredients in Anacin are: *(313)*
    1. acetaminophen and aspirin.
    2. aspirin and hydrocodone.
    3. acetaminophen and caffeine.
    4. aspirin and caffeine.
27. The nurse is instructing a patient who is allergic to acetaminophen (Tylenol) on the use of which combination product that would be safe to take? *(313)*
    1. Excedrin Extra Strength
    2. Fioricet
    3. Percocet 7.5
    4. Percodan

28. A nurse was explaining to the patient in the scenario the difference between Lortab and Vicodin, and states correctly: *(313)*
    1. "There is no difference; they are just made by different drug companies."
    2. "Lortab has more acetaminophen in it than Vicodin."
    3. "Lortab has more hydromorphone in it than Vicodin."
    4. "Lortab has more hydrocodone in it than Vicodin."

Identify opiate antagonists and expected therapeutic outcomes to monitor.

29. Emergency service personnel across the nation now carry the opiate antagonist naloxone (Evzio) for cases of: *(306)*
    1. acute anaphylaxis by bee stings.
    2. food poisoning.
    3. potential overdoses of opiates.
    4. acute hemorrhage.
30. By administering the opiate antagonist naloxone (Evzio), the nurse understands this drug is used to: *(Select all that apply.) (306)*
    1. reverse respiratory depression.
    2. increase GI motility.
    3. decrease the incidence of allergic reactions.
    4. reverse CNS depression caused by excessive doses of opiate agonists.
    5. block the euphoric high associated with pentazocine.
31. Which opiate antagonist can be given orally? *(307)*
    1. Naloxone
    2. Naltrexone
    3. Naproxen
    4. Nabumetone

Introduction to Cardiovascular Disease and Metabolic Syndrome

chapter

20

Answer Key: Textbook page references are provided as a guide for answering these questions. A complete answer key is provided to your instructor.

MATCHING

Match the term on the right with the definition on the left.

Definitions

1. _____ abnormalities in the electrical conduction pathways of the heart
2. _____ a narrowing or obstruction of the arteries of the heart
3. _____ an obstruction or rupture of blood vessels in the brain
4. _____ involves disorders of the blood vessels of the arms and legs
5. _____ an increase in the pressure with which blood circulates through the arteries

Terms

a. hypertension
b. dysrhythmias
c. coronary artery disease
d. peripheral vascular disease
e. stroke

REVIEW QUESTIONS

Scenario: A 42-year-old male patient discussed with the nurse the need for exercising, as he had previously indicated that he rarely exercises. The nurse was asking questions designed to get him to think about why he did not exercise and what some of his beliefs were about this, as he was obese and just diagnosed with hypertension.

Identify the major risk factors for the development of metabolic syndrome.

6. The nurse will explain to the patient in the scenario the risk factors that he needs to consider that may lead to the development of metabolic syndrome, which are: *(Select all that apply.)* *(318-320)*
   1. active lifestyle.
   2. stressful occupation.
   3. obesity.
   4. diabetes.
   5. hypertension.
7. The risk factor of lower levels of HDL cholesterol is important to consider for developing metabolic syndrome because it can lead to: *(318)*
   1. hypertension.
   2. diabetes.
   3. cardiovascular disorders.
   4. insulin resistance syndrome.
8. Examples of cardiovascular disorders that are attributed to the narrowing or obstruction of the arteries of the heart include: *(Select all that apply.)* *(317)*

   1. stroke.
   2. angina pectoris.
   3. myocardial infarction.
   4. hypertension.
   5. peripheral vascular disease.
9. In addition to type 2 diabetes and heart disease, which other consequences are associated with metabolic syndrome? *(Select all that apply.)* *(318)*
   1. Renal disease
   2. Liver disease
   3. Obstructive sleep apnea
   4. Cognitive decline in older adults
   5. Polycystic ovary syndrome
10. Examples of peripheral vascular disease involving disorders of the blood vessels of the arms and legs include: *(Select all that apply.)* *(317)*
    1. obstructive arterial disease.
    2. deep vein thrombosis.
    3. stroke.
    4. myocardial infarction.
    5. diabesity.

Discuss the importance of lifestyle modification in the management of metabolic syndrome.

11. Which factors should the nurse encourage when teaching health promotion to the patient in the scenario with metabolic syndrome? *(Select all that apply.)* *(320-321)*
    1. Smoking cessation
    2. Weight reduction

3. Vigorous exercise
4. Stress reduction
5. Dietary modification
12. When teaching the patient in the scenario about metabolic syndrome, the nurse discusses ways to promote weight loss and increased physical activity by which methods? *(Select all that apply.)* *(321)*
    1. Exercising at the same time of day consistently
    2. Reducing the number of calories eaten
    3. Getting 60 minutes of moderate-intensity physical activity twice a week
    4. Daily maximum caloric intake of food to be consumed based on age
    5. Adopting the DASH diet
13. Some of the contributing factors to a sedentary lifestyle that contribute to obesity and the development of metabolic syndrome include: *(Select all that apply.)* *(319)*
    1. remote control devices.
    2. genetic predisposition.
    3. entertainment through television and computers.
    4. labor-saving devices.
    5. work-related stress.

Explain the treatment goals for type 2 diabetes management, lipid management, and hypertension management.

14. Which drugs and/or drug classes are used to treat type 2 diabetes mellitus associated with metabolic syndrome because they will stimulate the beta cells of the pancreas to release more insulin? *(Select all that apply.)* *(321)*
    1. Sulfonylureas
    2. Metformin (Glucophage)
    3. Alpha-glycosidase (Acarbose)
    4. Meglitinides
    5. Thiazolidinediones
15. Treatment of dyslipidemia is generally to lower the triglycerides and LDL cholesterol and raise the HDL cholesterol and includes: *(Select all that apply.)* *(321)*
    1. calcium channel blockers.
    2. fibric acid derivatives.
    3. statins.
    4. alpha-glycosidase inhibitors.
    5. thiazide diuretics.

16. When teaching the patient in the scenario with metabolic syndrome about the importance of weight loss and a healthy diet, the nurse includes: *(320)*
    1. "Restrict the total amount of fat you consume each day to approximately 45% of your total calories."
    2. "You must limit the amount of protein you eat to 2 ounces once a day."
    3. "Most of the dietary fat you consume should be saturated."
    4. "Olive oil is an example of the type of 'good' fat you may eat."
17. The treatment for hypertension when changes in diet and exercise do not produce acceptable reduction in blood pressure include drug therapy such as: *(Select all that apply.)* *(321)*
    1. thiazide diuretics.
    2. angiotensin-converting enzyme inhibitors.
    3. analgesics.
    4. calcium channel blockers.
    5. alpha-glycosidase inhibitors.

Discuss the drug management of the underlying diseases used by patients with metabolic syndrome.

18. The overall treatment goals for metabolic syndrome include: *(Select all that apply.)* *(320)*
    1. triglyceride levels of < 150 mg/dL.
    2. hemoglobin A1C levels < 7%.
    3. fasting blood sugar of < 120 mg/dL.
    4. LDLs of < 100 mg/dL.
    5. blood pressure of < 150/90 mm Hg.
19. Managing metabolic syndrome will result in: *(Select all that apply.)* *(320)*
    1. increasing likelihood of developing diabetes.
    2. reduction in the development of cardiovascular diseases.
    3. reduction in the importance of genetic factors.
    4. improved management of obesity.
    5. reduction in insulin resistance.
20. Which lab values indicate that the general treatment goals for patients with metabolic syndrome are being met? *(Select all that apply.)* *(320)*
    1. LDLs of 140 mg/dL
    2. HDLs of 55 mg/dL
    3. Postprandial plasma glucose of of 140 mg/dL
    4. Hemoglobin A1C of 5%
    5. Fasting plasma glucose of 118 mg/dL

Drugs Used to Treat Dyslipidemias

chapter
21

Answer Key: Textbook page references are provided as a guide for answering these questions. A complete answer key is provided to your instructor.

MATCHING

Match the term on the right with the definition on the left.

Definition

1. _____ a cluster of risk factors that relate directly to excesses in lifestyle

2. _____ characterized by the accumulation of fatty deposits on the inner walls of blood vessels

3. _____ ninety percent triglycerides and five percent cholesterol

4. _____ an abnormal elevation of cholesterol and triglyceride levels in the blood

5. _____ a precursor of cholesterol

Term

a. hyperlipidemia
b. atherosclerosis
c. metabolic syndrome
d. triglycerides
e. chylomicrons

REVIEW QUESTIONS

Scenario: An obese 58-year-old female patient with hypertension and diabetes was told during a routine checkup that she had elevated levels of cholesterol and needed to be started on antilipid therapy along with diet modification.

Describe atherosclerosis and identify the four major types of lipoproteins.

6. Which condition is characterized by the accumulation of fatty deposits on the inner walls of arteries and arterioles throughout the body that reduce the blood supply to vital organs? *(323)*
    1. Myocardial infarction
    2. Atherosclerosis
    3. Angina pectoris
    4. Cardiac dysrhythmias

7. Major treatable causes of coronary artery disease (CAD) include: *(Select all that apply.) (323)*
    1. sedentary lifestyle.
    2. alcoholism.
    3. smoking.
    4. angina pectoris.
    5. type 2 diabetes.

8. Which lipoprotein is sometimes referred to as the "good" lipoprotein because high levels indicate that cholesterol is being removed from vascular tissue? *(323)*

    1. IDL
    2. VLDL
    3. LDL
    4. HDL

9. Atherosclerosis impacts the arteries of the heart as well as the arteries in the body, causing: *(323)*
    1. increased cerebral profusion.
    2. pulmonary hypotension.
    3. peripheral vascular disease.
    4. urinary retention.

10. Lipoproteins are subdivided into five categories based on composition: chylomicrons, very low-density lipoproteins (VLDLs), intermediate-density lipoproteins (IDLs), low-density lipoproteins (LDLs), and high-density lipoproteins (HDLs). The five types differ in concentration of: *(323)*
    1. cholesterol, triglycerides, and steroids.
    2. triglycerides, proteins, and amino acids.
    3. cholesterol, protein, and carbohydrates.
    4. triglycerides, cholesterol, and proteins.

11. Low levels of HDLs are considered a positive risk factor for the development of: *(324)*
    1. diabetes.
    2. bleeding disorders.
    3. coronary artery disease.
    4. elevated C-reactive protein levels.

Describe the primary approaches to treat lipid disorders.

12. The patient in the scenario came back to the clinic for a checkup after starting atorvastatin (Lipitor) and asked the nurse how the drug works. The best response by the nurse is: *(329)*
    1. "The statins work best when taken with another antilipid agent to lower your cholesterol level."
    2. "The statins inhibit an enzyme in the pathway to making cholesterol in the liver."
    3. "The exact action of statins is unknown, but they are effective agents in reducing cholesterol."
    4. "The statins interfere with the absorption of cholesterol from the diet."

13. Antilipid agents used to lower elevated cholesterol levels are the bile acid–binding resins and: *(Select all that apply.)* *(324)*
    1. niacin.
    2. omega-3 fatty acids.
    3. HMG-CoA reductase inhibitors.
    4. fibric acids.
    5. vitamin B_{12}.

14. Which antilipid agent reduces atherosclerosis by blocking the absorption of cholesterol by the small intestine? *(332)*
    1. Simvastatin
    2. Lovaza
    3. Ezetimibe
    4. Niacin

15. Which antilipid agent decreases atherosclerosis by combining two omega-3 fatty acids, which act to decrease the synthesis of triglycerides in the liver? *(333)*
    1. Ezetimibe
    2. Lovaza
    3. Atorvastatin
    4. Gemfibrozil

Determine which antilipid medications are used for cholesterol control and which can be used for triglyceride control.

16. Antilipid agents are used to treat hyperlipidemias only if attempts to lower LDL-C levels by which means are not successful? *(Select all that apply.)* *(324)*
    1. Weight reduction
    2. Diet low in cholesterol and fat
    3. Increasing vitamin intake
    4. Exercise
    5. Improved hand hygiene

17. The statins are the most potent antilipid agents available with which added benefits that result in decreased heart attacks and stroke? *(Select all that apply.)* *(329)*
    1. Decreased amounts of HDL
    2. Decreased inflammation
    3. Decreased platelet aggregation
    4. Decreased thrombin formation
    5. Decreased plasma viscosity

18. Which antilipid agents are used to reduce triglyceride levels for patients who have hypertriglyceridemia? *(Select all that apply.)* *(324)*
    1. Niacin
    2. Omega-3 fatty acids
    3. Fibric acids
    4. Statins
    5. Bile acid–binding resins

Differentiate between how statins work to control lipid levels and how the bile acid resins work to control lipid levels.

19. The nurse instructing the patient in the scenario taking a HMG-CoA reductase inhibitor for the treatment of hyperlipidemia, reminded her to: *(331)*
    1. avoid grapefruit juice.
    2. increase any anticoagulants taken by twice as much.
    3. expect muscle weakness as a common adverse effect.
    4. take the medication on an empty stomach to increase absorption.

20. When teaching a patient about niacin therapy, the nurse tells the patient to report which adverse effects to the primary healthcare provider? *(Select all that apply.)* *(329)*
    1. Flushing
    2. Tingling
    3. Fatigue
    4. Muscle aches
    5. Jaundice

21. A patient taking a bile acid–binding resin for the treatment of dyslipidemia tells the nurse that ever since he began taking the medication, he experiences bloating and fullness. What does the nurse instruct the patient to do? *(Select all that apply.)* *(328)*
    1. Swallow the medication without gulping air.
    2. Maintain adequate fiber in the diet.
    3. Limit fluid intake.
    4. Take the medication with a carbonated beverage.
    5. Use a daily laxative.

Drugs Used to Treat Hypertension

Answer Key: Textbook page references are provided as a guide for answering these questions. A complete answer key is provided to your instructor.

MATCHING

Match the drug classification on the right with the drug name on the left. Classifications may be used more than once.

Drug Name	Drug Classification
1. _____ candesartan	a. beta blockers
2. _____ ramipril	b. diuretics
3. _____ metoprolol	c. angiotensin-converting enzyme inhibitors
4. _____ aliskiren	d. angiotensin II receptor blockers
5. _____ hydralazine	e. calcium channel blockers
6. _____ doxazosin	f. direct vasodilators
7. _____ eplerenone	g. aldosterone receptor antagonist
8. _____ valsartan	h. renin inhibitor
9. _____ spironolactone	i. alpha-1 adrenergic blocking agents
10. _____ atenolol	j. central-acting alpha-2 agonists
11. _____ lisinopril	
12. _____ clonidine	
13. _____ amlodipine	
14. _____ hydrochlorothiazide	
15. _____ verapamil	

REVIEW QUESTIONS

Scenario: A 42-year-old man came into the clinic complaining of frequent headaches and was diagnosed with stage 1 hypertension. He was referred to the education specialist for further instructions on lifestyle modification and initiation of drug therapy.

Differentiate between primary and secondary hypertension.

16. A patient has a blood pressure reading of 170/102 mm Hg. The nurse identifies this patient as having which classification of hypertension? *(337)*
    1. Normal
    2. Prehypertension
    3. Stage 1
    4. Stage 2

17. A nurse was discussing the difference between primary and secondary hypertension with the patient in the scenario. The best explanation that should be given is: *(336)*
    1. "Primary hypertension occurs during adolescence, while secondary hypertension happens to people after they reach adulthood."
    2. "There is no difference between primary and secondary hypertension; both of them can be cured."
    3. "Primary hypertension occurs about 90% of the time and has no known cause, while secondary occurs after the development of another disorder."
    4. "Primary hypertension is curable, while secondary hypertension is only controllable."

18. Which conditions are identifiable causes of hypertension? *(Select all that apply.)* *(336)*
    1. Sleep apnea
    2. Chronic kidney disease
    3. Primary aldosteronism
    4. Marfan's syndrome
    5. Thyroid disease
19. Various types of antihypertensive agents have an effect on the system that plays an important role in the development of hypertension, known as the: *(346)*
    1. RAAS cascade.
    2. coagulation cascade.
    3. CIWA scale.
    4. adrenergic blocking system.

Summarize nursing assessments and interventions used for the treatment of hypertension.

20. What will the nurse do to measure a patient's blood pressure? *(Select all that apply.)* *(342)*
    1. Use an appropriate-sized cuff.
    2. Verify reading in the opposite arm.
    3. Sit the patient in a chair with feet dangling off the floor.
    4. Wait at least 5 minutes before measuring the blood pressure.
    5. Support the arm at the same level as the heart.
21. Which drug class includes the most commonly prescribed antihypertensive agents? *(344)*
    1. Diuretics
    2. ACE inhibitors
    3. Angiotensin II receptor blockers
    4. Calcium channel blockers
22. For patients who are diagnosed with hypertension, further evaluation must be obtained that includes: *(Select all that apply.)* *(337)*
    1. physical exam.
    2. any history of tonsillectomy or appendectomy.
    3. any presence of target organ damage.
    4. current understanding of the drugs used for hypertension.
    5. laboratory tests to identify possible causes of hypertension.
23. Systolic blood pressure is the pressure exerted by the heart as blood is pumped out; diastolic blood pressure is the pressure present: *(335)*
    1. during the peak of physical activity.
    2. after the blood returns to the heart.
    3. during the resting phase of the heartbeat.
    4. when the valves of the heart close.
24. The nurse needs to monitor the patient in the scenario for any changes in mental status, muscle strength, muscle cramps, tremors, or nausea because these are signs of: *(349)*
    1. orthostatic hypotension.
    2. hepatotoxicity.
    3. depression.
    4. electrolyte imbalance.

25. The purpose of controlling hypertension is to reduce the frequency of which disorders? *(Select all that apply.)* *(337)*
    1. Hyperthyroidism
    2. Bladder cancer
    3. Stroke
    4. Renal failure
    5. Cardiovascular disease

Identify recommended lifestyle modifications after a diagnosis of hypertension.

26. When discussing the modifications that are recommended for the patient in the scenario, the nurse will review: *(Select all that apply.)* *(343)*
    1. using the DASH diet.
    2. over-the-counter diet aids.
    3. weight reduction.
    4. maintaining usual sodium intake.
    5. moderate to heavy physical activity 5 times a week.
27. The nutritional goals for the treatment of hypertension include: *(Select all that apply.)* *(337)*
    1. limit consumption of alcohol to no more than two drinks per day.
    2. reduce the amount of dietary sodium intake.
    3. eat more fruits and vegetables.
    4. consume more dairy products per day.
    5. reduce the amount of water consumed to prevent renal damage.
28. A patient asks the nurse how much exercise is considered enough for the control of blood pressure. The nurse knows that a range of 4-9 mm Hg of approximate systolic pressure reduction can occur with engaging in regular physical activity: *(338)*
    1. for only 3 days a week.
    2. at least 40 minutes per session.
    3. at the most, 15-20 minutes a week.
    4. for as little as 90 minutes a week.
29. The nurse was instructing the patient in the scenario regarding lifestyle modification and recognized that further education was needed after the patient made which statement? *(337)*
    1. "I know that I will have to stop eating tortilla chips since they have a lot of salt."
    2. "So my plan is to start losing weight gradually so I can keep it off."
    3. "I understand that I need to walk more than just twice a week, so I think I will walk four times a week."
    4. "Since I will be started on drug therapy for my high blood pressure, I do not need to change my habits."

Identify initial options and progression of medicines used to treat hypertension (see Figure 22-2).

30. The nurse expects that the patient in the scenario may be started on: *(Select all that apply.)* *(338)*
    1. diuretics.

2. angiotensin-converting enzyme inhibitors.
3. calcium channel blockers.
4. aldosterone receptor antagonists.
5. beta blockers.

31. After being on a thiazide for several months, a patient being treated for stage 1 hypertension will most likely have which medication added because the target blood pressure was not attained? *(338-339)*
    1. Aliskiren (Tekturna)
    2. Eplerenone (Inspra)
    3. Nifedipine (Procardia)
    4. Spironolactone (Aldactone)

32. For patients who have stage 2 hypertension and need to be started on two-drug combinations for blood pressure control, which drug classes may be started? *(Select all that apply.)* *(340)*
    1. Diuretics
    2. Renin inhibitors
    3. Angiotensin II receptor blockers statins
    4. Calcium channel blockers
    5. Angiotensin-converting enzyme inhibitors

33. The patient in the scenario asks the nurse about risk factors for developing hypertension and the nurse's response includes: *(Select all that apply.)* *(337)*
    1. "The risk factors that cannot be managed are your age, gender, and race."
    2. "The best way to treat high blood pressure is to limit your salt intake."
    3. "With exercise and proper diet, you can start to help manage your blood pressure."
    4. "Lifestyle changes are important to recognize as part of the management of hypertension."
    5. "You will need to get a low-stress job since that is the best way to manage your high blood pressure."

34. While discussing the best way to change diet habits with a patient who has hypertension, the nurse asks: *(342)*
    1. the patient to estimate the percentage of total daily calories from fats.
    2. how foods are prepared, as fried foods are preferred over baked or broiled.
    3. the portion size and number of servings the patient eats of meat, fish, and poultry.
    4. the patient to restrict the amount of dairy products in the diet.

35. A patient in the scenario was discussing how to manage his blood pressure with the nurse and mentioned that he likes to smoke an occasional cigar. What is the best response from the nurse? *(343)*

1. "That should be okay; smoking does not affect your blood pressure."
2. "You will need to stop smoking altogether, since that is very bad for you."
3. "How often would you say is 'occasional'?"
4. "Did you know that smoking will cause the diuretic you are on to be ineffective?"

Identify and summarize the action of five drug classes used to treat hypertension.

36. Which drugs are direct vasodilators? *(Select all that apply.)* *(360)*
    1. Methyldopa
    2. Nitroprusside sodium (Nitropress)
    3. Guanadrel (Hylorel)
    4. Hydralazine (Apresoline)
    5. Aliskiren (Tekturna)

37. Which class of antihypertensive agents lowers blood pressure by blocking a very potent vasoconstrictor from binding to the receptor sites in vascular smooth muscle, brain, heart, kidneys, and adrenal glands? *(345)*
    1. Beta blockers
    2. Angiotensin II receptor blockers
    3. Calcium channel blockers
    4. Aldosterone receptor antagonists

38. If patients develop a chronic, dry, nonproductive cough and are taking which antihypertensive agent, they will need to contact their healthcare provider to get a different agent? *(348)*
    1. Metoprolol
    2. Hydralazine
    3. Captopril
    4. Amlodipine

39. Calcium channel blockers are used for the reduction of blood pressure and: *(Select all that apply.)* *(354)*
    1. peripheral vasodilating effects.
    2. reducing afterload.
    3. increasing sodium excretion.
    4. increasing preload.
    5. peripheral vasoconstricting effects.

40. The drug prazosin, an alpha-1 adrenergic blocking agent, has which therapeutic outcomes? *(Select all that apply.)* *(357)*
    1. Reducing blood lipids
    2. Improving urine flow
    3. Reducing gastric acid production
    4. Reducing blood pressure
    5. Improving memory

Drugs Used to Treat Dysrhythmias

Answer Key: Textbook page references are provided as a guide for answering these questions. A complete answer key is provided to your instructor.

MATCHING

Match the drug classification on the right with the drug name on the left. Classifications may be used more than once.

	Drug Name		Drug Classification
1.	_____ dofetilide	a.	class Ia
2.	_____ propafenone	b.	class Ib
3.	_____ quinidine	c.	class Ic
4.	_____ disopyramide	d.	class II
5.	_____ flecainide	e.	class III
6.	_____ esmolol		
7.	_____ amiodarone		
8.	_____ lidocaine		

REVIEW QUESTIONS

Scenario: An 89-year-old male patient was admitted to the hospital after falling and fracturing his arm. He has a history of atrial fibrillation and had a permanent pacemaker implanted several years ago.

Describe the anatomic structures and conduction system of the heart.

9. The conduction system of the heart begins in the pacemaker cells known as the: *(363)*
   1. bundle of His.
   2. atrioventricular (AV) node.
   3. sinoatrial (SA) node.
   4. Purkinje fibers.
10. Identify the sequence of the electrical current as it travels through the conduction system of the heart in the correct order. *(363)*
    1. _____ Purkinje fibers
    2. _____ AV node
    3. _____ Bundle of His
    4. _____ SA node
11. When the electrical current passes through the SA node, it causes the: *(363)*
    1. ventricles to contract.
    2. atrial muscle to contract and fill the ventricles.

3. blood to be pumped out through the aorta.
4. heart muscle to contract from the apex.

12. Dysrhythmias may be caused by abnormal pacemaker cells, as well as: *(363)*
    1. a blockage of the normal electrical pathways.
    2. a contraction of the atrial muscle.
    3. an opening in the Purkinje fibers.
    4. the flow of blood through the SA node.
13. Dysrhythmias that develop above the bundle of His are called *supraventricular dysrhythmias*, and include: *(Select all that apply.)* *(364)*
    1. sinus bradycardia.
    2. atrial flutter/atrial fibrillation.
    3. normal sinus rhythm.
    4. premature atrial contractions.
    5. paroxysmal supraventricular tachycardia.
14. Dysrhythmias that develop below the bundle of His are referred to as *ventricular dysrhythmias* and include: *(Select all that apply.)* *(364)*
    1. sinus tachycardia.
    2. premature ventricular contractions.
    3. ventricular tachycardia.
    4. ventricular fibrillation.
    5. atrial tachycardia.

Identify the classification of drugs used to treat dysrhythmias.

15. The goal of treatment for dysrhythmias is to restore normal sinus rhythm and: *(364)*
    1. speed up the rate of the heart.
    2. increase the contractility of the heart muscle.
    3. improve the output from the atrial muscle.
    4. prevent recurrence of life-threatening dysrhythmias.

16. Of the medications that the patient in the scenario is taking, the nurse recognizes which medication for the treatment of atrial fibrillation? *(376)*
    1. Irbesartan (Avapro)
    2. Tramadol (Ultram)
    3. Omeprazole (Prilosec)
    4. Digoxin (Lanoxin)

17. Which class of antidysrhythmics acts as myocardial depressants by inhibiting sodium ion movement of the heart? *(365)*
    1. Class I agents
    2. Class II agents
    3. Class III agents
    4. Class IV agents

18. Which class of antidysrhythmic drugs is effective in inhibiting cardiac response to sympathetic nerve stimulation, and as a result reduces heart rate, blood pressure, and cardiac output? *(371)*
    1. Calcium channel blockers
    2. Beta-adrenergic blockers
    3. Potassium channel blockers
    4. Sodium channel blockers

Identify baseline nursing assessments that should be implemented during the treatment of dysrhythmias.

19. Which methods are used to assess dysrhythmias that patients develop? *(Select all that apply.)* *(366)*
    1. Electric shock therapy
    2. Exercise electrocardiography
    3. Electrocardiogram (ECG) monitoring
    4. Electrophysiologic studies (EPS)
    5. Laboratory values

20. The nurse recognizes that it is important to monitor the hourly urine output in a patient with dysrhythmias because this will: *(366)*
    1. indicate the function of the atrial muscle.
    2. determine the cardiac output.
    3. reflect whether the kidney tissues are being adequately perfused.
    4. reflect the perfusion of the peripheral tissues.

21. Assessing a cardiac patient for level of consciousness is one of the important baseline assessments that the nurse will perform to determine adequate: *(366)*
    1. peripheral perfusion.
    2. cerebral tissue perfusion.
    3. renal perfusion.
    4. lung perfusion.

22. When given intravenously, amiodarone needs to be administered: *(372)*
    1. slowly over an hour, and flushed immediately.
    2. slowly over an hour, then followed with a continuous drip.
    3. quickly over 10 minutes, then flushed immediately.
    4. quickly over 10 minutes, then followed with a continuous drip.

23. The nurse needs to monitor which vital signs of patients who are taking antidysrhythmic drugs? *(Select all that apply.)* *(366)*
    1. Blood pressure in both arms
    2. Pulse quality
    3. Adequate output
    4. Respirations
    5. Oxygen saturation

24. The laboratory tests that should be monitored for patients taking antidysrhythmic drugs include: *(Select all that apply.)* *(366)*
    1. electrolytes.
    2. arterial blood gases.
    3. creatine kinase (CK-MB).
    4. thyroid levels.
    5. gastric pH.

Cite common adverse effects that may be observed with the administration of antidysrhythmic drugs.

25. Amiodarone may cause serious adverse effects and because of this, the patient will need periodic tests for: *(Select all that apply.)* *(372-373)*
    1. thyroid function.
    2. visual disturbance.
    3. liver function.
    4. pulmonary function.
    5. hearing loss.

26. The nurse is teaching the patient in the scenario that he will be started on propafenone (Rythmol) for further control of his atrial fibrillation. The nurse teaches him to be alert for common adverse effects of the drug including: *(Select all that apply.)* *(371)*
    1. nausea and vomiting.
    2. constipation.
    3. sleep disturbances.
    4. tremors.
    5. dizziness.

27. Caution must be taken with patients who receive a neuromuscular blockade while also receiving quinidine because: *(369)*
    1. quinidine will increase bleeding time.
    2. quinidine may prolong the effects of these muscle relaxants.
    3. respiratory muscles are stimulated with quinidine.
    4. CNS response to quinidine causes lethargy.

28. When assessing the patient who is taking quinidine, following the administration of succinylcholine for a biopsy, the nurse observes for signs of: *(369)*

   1.   bleeding gums and bruises.
   2.   anorexia, nausea, and vomiting.
   3.   respiratory depression.
   4.   tinnitus.

List the six cardinal signs of cardiovascular disease.

29. The cardinal sign of cardiovascular disease that involves the respiratory system is: *(365-366)*
   1.   dyspnea.
   2.   palpitation.
   3.   edema.
   4.   syncope.

30. The patient in the scenario began to feel tired easily and starting to take naps in the afternoon. Which sign of cardiovascular disease does this represent? *(365-366)*
   1.   Chest pain
   2.   Fatigue
   3.   Edema
   4.   Syncope

31. When monitoring patients for signs of cardiovascular disease, the nurse will observe for edema. Where are the specific areas in the body most likely to show signs of edema? *(Select all that apply.)* *(366)*
   1.   Arms
   2.   Mid-calf
   3.   Ankles
   4.   Thigh
   5.   Hands

32. The patient in the scenario told the nurse that he felt as though his heart was skipping some beats. The nurse recognized this symptom as which one of the six cardinal signs of cardiovascular disease? *(366)*
   1.   Dyspnea
   2.   Syncope
   3.   Fatigue
   4.   Palpitations

Drugs Used to Treat Angina Pectoris

chapter

24

Answer Key: Textbook page references are provided as a guide for answering these questions. A complete answer key is provided to your instructor.

MATCHING
Match the term on the right with the definition on the left.

Definition

1. _____ occurs while the patient is at rest, caused by vasospasms of the coronary artery, diagnosed by combination of history and exercise testing

2. _____ precipitated by physical exertion or stress, lasts only a few minutes, relieved by nitroglycerin

3. _____ unpredictable; changes in onset, frequency, duration, and intensity

4. _____ supply of oxygen needed by the heart cells is inadequate

5. _____ feeling of chest discomfort arising from the heart

Term

a. unstable angina
b. ischemia
c. chronic stable angina
d. angina pectoris
e. variant angina

REVIEW QUESTIONS

Scenario: A 52-year-old male patient was admitted through the emergency department to a telemetry unit after experiencing sudden substernal chest pain radiating down his left arm, feeling faint, and indigestion. He was a history of urinary retention, palpitations, insomnia, and depression.

Define *angina pectoris* and identify assessment data needed to evaluate an anginal attack.

6. The underlying cause of anginal pain is a result of: *(379)*
   1. a cardiac dysrhythmia.
   2. the lack of an adequate oxygen supply to the cells in the heart.
   3. decreased circulation to the chest muscles.
   4. a severe increase in blood pressure.

7. The patient in the scenario has various presenting symptoms of angina (in addition to the substernal chest pain radiating down his left arm), which include: *(Select all that apply.) (381)*
   1. palpitations.
   2. depression.
   3. urinary retention.
   4. feeling faint.
   5. insomnia.

8. The nurse needs to gather which assessment data from patients who present with angina? *(Select all that apply.) (381)*
   1. What medications are being taken
   2. The degree of understanding regarding lifestyle modifications
   3. Vital signs and pulse checks
   4. Any smoking history
   5. The onset, duration, and intensity of pain

Differentiate between *chronic stable angina* and *unstable angina* and the drug therapy used for each type.

9. The patient in the scenario is considered to have which type of angina? *(379)*
   1. Variant angina
   2. Unstable angina
   3. Chronic angina
   4. Stable angina

10. The difference between unstable angina and chronic stable angina is: *(379)*
    1. chronic angina is relieved with rest and unstable angina is relieved with exercise.
    2. unstable angina is caused by vasospasm and chronic angina is caused by a fixed obstruction.
    3. chronic angina is unpredictable in nature and unstable angina occurs at regular intervals.

4. unstable angina is relieved with nitroglycerin and chronic angina is relieved with statin drugs.

11. The nurse was explaining to the patient in the scenario the treatment goals for angina and included in the discussion: *(Select all that apply.)* *(379)*
    1. "The choices you have for treatment therapies are designed to prevent a heart attack."
    2. "Your healthcare team wants to improve quality of life by relieving your anginal pain."
    3. "You may have the choice of either angioplasty or bypass surgery depending on the results of further tests."
    4. "Depending on the results of your tests, you will be instructed to make changes in your lifestyle prior to starting on any drug therapy."
    5. "In the future when you have anginal pain, you can take a Tylenol first before taking any nitroglycerin."

12. Premedication assessments that the nurse should perform prior to initiating therapy with nitrates for patients with heart disease include: *(Select all that apply.)* *(383)*
    1. checking laboratory results of HDLs.
    2. the ability to place the medication under the tongue correctly.
    3. pain assessment.
    4. most recent nitrate use.
    5. any history of gastritis.

Describe the actions of nitrates, beta-adrenergic blockers, calcium channel blockers, and angiotensin-converting enzyme inhibitors on the myocardial tissue of the heart.

13. The desired action of calcium channel blockers in the treatment of angina is to: *(Select all that apply.)* *(387)*
    1. decrease the workload of the heart.
    2. decrease resistance to blood flow.
    3. increase myocardial blood supply via coronary arteries.
    4. dilate the peripheral blood vessels.
    5. decrease the peripheral circulation.

14. The common adverse effects associated with angiotensin-converting enzyme inhibitors include: *(Select all that apply.)* *(388)*
    1. nasal congestion.
    2. hypotension with dizziness.
    3. fainting.
    4. tachycardia.
    5. indigestion or heartburn.

15. Patients with a history of which disorder are at the highest risk for complications associated with use of beta-adrenergic blockers for the treatment of angina? *(386)*
    1. High blood pressure
    2. Gastric ulcer
    3. Anemia
    4. Respiratory disorders

16. Nitrates are used for therapy to treat angina because they: *(382)*
    1. increase the serum creatinine.
    2. cause blood vessels to dilate, allowing more blood flow.
    3. prevent platelet aggregation.
    4. lower the amount of circulating LDLs.

17. ACE inhibitors are effective in relieving anginal attacks because they: *(388)*
    1. prolong the QT interval.
    2. lower the amount of circulating LDLs.
    3. promote vasodilation and minimize platelet aggregation.
    4. decrease serum creatinine.

18. Calcium channel blockers are used to relieve anginal attacks because they: *(387)*
    1. lower the amount of circulating LDLs.
    2. prevent platelet aggregation.
    3. increase calcium levels in the blood.
    4. dilate the peripheral vessels and inhibit smooth muscle contractions.

19. Common adverse effects of nitrate therapy are: *(Select all that apply.)* *(385-386)*
    1. excessive hypotension.
    2. tolerance.
    3. nausea.
    4. prolonged headache.
    5. bradycardia.

20. The nurse includes which statements when teaching a patient about the use of nitroglycerin spray (Nitrolingual)? *(Select all that apply.)* *(383)*
    1. "Do not shake the container before administration."
    2. "Hold the canister vertically when administering the medication."
    3. "Spray the dose onto the roof of your mouth."
    4. "Do not inhale or swallow the spray."
    5. "Call 911 if chest pain is not relieved by one dose within 5 minutes."

Identify risk factor management and healthy lifestyle changes that are taught to prevent disease progression and myocardial infarction or death.

21. The nurse will teach a patient to do what at the first sign of an anginal attack? *(381)*
    1. Call 911.
    2. Sit or lie down.
    3. Take two nitroglycerin tablets.
    4. Take an extra dose of transdermal nitroglycerin.

22. In addition to weight control and a structured exercise program, the nurse should also educate the patient on other ways of improving cardiovascular health such as managing which conditions? *(Select all that apply.)* *(382)*
    1. Dyslipidemia
    2. Hypothyroidism
    3. Hypertension
    4. Diabetes mellitus
    5. Migraines

23. The nurse was explaining to the patient in the scenario about the need to avoid activities that precipitate attacks of angina, which may include: *(Select all that apply.)* **(380)**
    1. eating a light lunch.
    2. exposure to cold temperatures.
    3. watching TV.
    4. climbing a flight of stairs.
    5. lifting heavy boxes.

Drugs Used to Treat Peripheral Vascular Disease

Answer Key: Textbook page references are provided as a guide for answering these questions. A complete answer key is provided to your instructor.

MATCHING

Match the term on the right with the definition on the left.

Definition		Term
1. _____	a condition caused by vasospasms of the blood vessels triggered by unknown mechanisms	a. arteriosclerosis obliterans
2. _____	numbness with a tingling sensation	b. intermittent claudication
3. _____	vasoconstriction of blood vessels	c. paresthesias
4. _____	pain secondary to lack of oxygen to the muscles during exercise	d. Raynaud's disease
5. _____	obstructive arterial disease resulting from atherosclerotic plaque formation	e. vasospasm

REVIEW QUESTIONS

Scenario: An 81-year-old male patient was admitted to the hospital with complaints of progressive pain in both legs with activity that no longer goes away when the activity is stopped.

Describe the baseline assessments needed to evaluate a patient with peripheral vascular disease.

6. The nurse needs to assess for what after patients are started on vasodilating agents? *(395)*
   1. Orthostatic hypotension
   2. Pulsus paradoxus
   3. Paresthesias
   4. Thrombus formation
7. The most common form of peripheral vascular disease is: *(391)*
   1. arteritis.
   2. arteriosclerosis obliterans.
   3. Raynaud's disease.
   4. coarctation of the aorta.
8. Baseline assessments the nurse will gather on the patient in the scenario regarding peripheral vascular disease include: *(Select all that apply.) (393)*
   1. skin temperature.
   2. peripheral pulses.
   3. limb pain.
   4. presence of edema.
   5. respiratory rate.

9. The patient in the scenario has symptoms that may indicate intermittent claudication that is progressing. The nurse would expect which findings as further evidence of arteriosclerosis? *(Select all that apply.) (391)*
   1. Warmer skin temperature of the legs
   2. Poor pulses in the feet
   3. Cooler skin temperature of the legs
   4. Paresthesias
   5. Pink-colored skin
10. The phrase *peripheral vascular disease* can be applied to a variety of disorders and illnesses such as: *(Select all that apply.) (391)*
    1. arterial disease affecting the extremities.
    2. coronary heart disease.
    3. venous obstructions caused by thrombosis.
    4. arterial spasms.
    5. aortic stenosis.

Identify specific measures that the patient can use to improve peripheral circulation and prevent the complications of peripheral vascular disease.

11. Major treatable causes of peripheral vascular disease include: *(Select all that apply.) (392)*
    1. cigarette smoking.
    2. hypertension.
    3. diet high in antioxidants.
    4. atherosclerosis.
    5. aortic stenosis.

12. Without specific orders to do so from the healthcare provider, patients with peripheral vascular disease should be taught not to elevate their extremities above the level of the: *(394)*
    1. bladder.
    2. heart.
    3. liver.
    4. eyes.

13. The most cost-effective and successful forms of treatment for peripheral vascular disease are: *(Select all that apply.)* *(392)*
    1. weight reduction.
    2. smoking cessation.
    3. dietary modification.
    4. exercise.
    5. medications.

Identify the systemic effects to expect when peripheral vasodilating agents are administered.

14. The nurse teaching self-assessment to the patient in the scenario advises which measures to promote tissue perfusion? *(Select all that apply.)* *(394)*
    1. Reduce and stop smoking.
    2. Wear constricting stockings.
    3. Elevate the extremities when sitting.
    4. Elevate the head of the bed.
    5. Visually inspect the feet to note any skin breakdown.

15. Which agent used for treatment of intermittent claudication is thought to work by increasing erythrocyte flexibility? *(395)*
    1. Pentoxifylline (Trental)
    2. Adenosine (Adenocard)
    3. Cilostazol (Pletal)
    4. verapamil (Calan)

16. Classes of drugs that have been used successfully for the treatment of Raynaud's disease include: *(Select all that apply.)* *(392)*
    1. direct vasodilators.
    2. calcium channel blockers.
    3. adrenergic antagonists.
    4. angiotensin-converting enzyme inhibitors.
    5. sodium channel blockers.

17. The nurse collecting assessment data on the patient in the scenario for evidence of circulatory impairment in his legs needs to include: *(Select all that apply.)* *(393-394)*
    1. checking the pedal and radial pulses.
    2. asking about the frequency and volume of alcoholic beverages consumed.
    3. determining the number of cigarettes or cigars smoked daily.
    4. comparing the pulses in the extremities.
    5. using a Doppler ultrasound to help determine peripheral blood flow.

Explain why hypotension and tachycardia occur frequently with the use of peripheral vasodilators.

18. Nitroglycerin ointment was used as a treatment for Raynaud's disease, but which adverse effects limit its use? *(Select all that apply.)* *(392)*
    1. Dizziness
    2. Headache
    3. Numbness and tingling of hands
    4. Postural hypotension
    5. Intermittent claudication

19. Because certain medications used for the treatment of peripheral vascular disease cause vasodilation, the nurse will need to instruct the patient to: *(395)*
    1. drink four glasses of water daily.
    2. cross her legs when sitting.
    3. encourage a diet high in salt intake.
    4. rise slowly.

20. Instructions for an individual with peripheral vascular disease should include: *(395)*
    1. medical treatment from a healthcare provider.
    2. yearly dental checkups.
    3. regular trimming of toenails and corns.
    4. annual flu vaccine.

21. The nurse will include which statement when teaching a patient about pentoxifylline (Trental) for treatment of peripheral vascular disease? *(396)*
    1. "You will need to have a blood test called an INR to monitor the effects of this drug."
    2. "This drug must be taken on an empty stomach."
    3. "This drug may cause your blood pressure to be lower."
    4. "If this drug makes you feel dizzy, stop taking it immediately."

22. When are vasodilators used for the treatment of Reynaud's disease? *(392)*
    1. When the collateral circulation has improved.
    2. When blanching of the fingers and toes occurs.
    3. When the disease interferes with the ability to work.
    4. When the disease has progressed and a thrombus is present.

Cite both pharmacologic and nonpharmacologic goals of the treatment for peripheral vascular disease.

23. The nurse was discussing with the patient some of the options that the healthcare provider and patient had reviewed earlier in the day. To clarify the patient's options, the nurse could make which therapeutic statement? *(395)*
    1. "The provider talked to you about surgical options when you feel the medications are no longer effective."
    2. "The surgical options are the way to go and get this problem taken care of, in my opinion."
    3. "The provider said to you that amputation of your leg is the next step, rather than angioplasty or bypass grafting."

4. "There is nothing further we can do for you. You will just have to suffer because there are no more options available to you other than the medications."

24. Which two agents are the only ones approved by the FDA for treatment of intermittent claudication caused by occlusive arterial disease? *(392)*
    1. Clopidogrel and vorapaxar
    2. Verapamil and nifedipine
    3. Pentoxifylline and cilostazol
    4. Papaverine and isoxsuprine

25. A patient asks the nurse what can be done to decrease the occurrence and severity of vasospastic attacks of Raynaud's disease. How does the nurse respond? *(Select all that apply.)* *(392)*

1. "Most attacks of Raynaud's disease can be stopped by avoiding hot temperatures."
2. "Tobacco use is highly associated with vasospastic attacks of Raynaud's disease."
3. "It is not known what really triggers the vasospastic attacks seen with Raynaud's disease."
4. "The signs and symptoms associated with Raynaud's disease are due to vasospasm of the arteries of the skin of the hands, fingers, and sometimes toes."
5. "Most people have Raynaud's disease for a few years and then it goes away."

Drugs Used to Treat Thromboembolic Disorders

chapter
26

Answer Key: Textbook page references are provided as a guide for answering these questions. A complete answer key is provided to your instructor.

MATCHING
Match the drug class on the right with the drug name on the left. Drug classes may be used more than once.

	Drug Name		**Drug Class**
1.	_____ alteplase	a.	platelet inhibitors
2.	_____ apixaban	b.	anticoagulants
3.	_____ aspirin	c.	thrombin inhibitors
4.	_____ clopidogrel	d.	fibrinolytic agents
5.	_____ coumadin	e.	glycoprotein IIb/IIIa inhibitors
6.	_____ dabigatran		
7.	_____ dalteparin		
8.	_____ dipyridamole		
9.	_____ eptifibatide		
10.	_____ heparin		

REVIEW QUESTIONS

Scenario: An 82-year-old woman who was admitted to the hospital with a stroke has a history of atrial fibrillation and noncompliance with medications.

Explain the primary purposes of anticoagulant therapy.

11. Anticoagulant therapy is for patients who have which conditions? *(Select all that apply.)* *(400)*
    1. Myocardial infarction
    2. Deep vein thrombosis
    3. Pulmonary embolism
    4. Claudication
    5. Anemia
12. Which factors trigger blood clot formation? *(Select all that apply.)* *(399)*
    1. Circulating clotting proteins
    2. Fibrinogen activated by thrombin to soluble fibrin
    3. Damage to a blood vessel wall

    4. The presence of potassium in the cells
    5. Increased blood viscosity
13. When patients are placed on anticoagulants, the effect on the blood clot is that it: *(401)*
    1. becomes trapped in a capillary.
    2. is prevented from growing.
    3. circulates throughout the bloodstream.
    4. is dissolved.
14. What is the difference between red and white blood clots? *(399-400)*
    1. Red clots are fragile and break easily; white clots are stationary.
    2. Red clots are made up of platelets and fibrin; white clots are made of fibrin and erythrocytes.
    3. Red clots develop in arteries; white clots develop in veins.
    4. Red clots are made up of fibrin and erythrocytes; white clots are made of platelets and fibrin.

Describe conditions that place an individual at risk for developing blood clots and nursing interventions used to prevent these conditions.

15. Which conditions put patients at risk for developing blood clots? *(Select all that apply.)* *(399)*
    1. Heart failure
    2. Certain types of cancers
    3. Immobilization or trauma of the lower limbs
    4. Eating large amounts of green leafy vegetables
    5. Pregnancy and oral contraceptives
16. The patient in the scenario was at risk for developing a clot that breaks off and creates a pulmonary embolism because: *(Select all that apply.)* *(401)*
    1. there was noncompliance with her medications.
    2. she was taking her medications on a regular basis.
    3. she had atrial fibrillation, which is known to cause blood clots.
    4. she walked slowly because of her advanced age and it slowed her blood flow.
    5. the healthcare provider had not prescribed the correct medications to prevent a stroke.
17. What nursing actions can help prevent the formation of a clot in those patients who are at risk for developing blood clots? *(Select all that apply.)* *(401)*
    1. Apply sequential compression devices as ordered by the healthcare provider.
    2. Assess perfusion of extremities.
    3. Restrict fluid intake to 1 liter/day.
    4. Review lab data such as hematocrit and platelet count.
    5. Flex the patient's knees when on bed rest.
18. The nurse was teaching a patient about nutrition related to warfarin (Coumadin) therapy, and the nurse will include which statements in the patient education? *(Select all that apply.)* *(415)*
    1. "Limit intake of green leafy vegetables."
    2. "Drink six to eight 8-ounce glasses of water daily."
    3. "Carrots are to be excluded from your diet."
    4. "You must not eat more than one serving of protein a day."
    5. "Avoid foods that contain potassium."

Identify the actions of platelet inhibitors, anticoagulants, thrombin inhibitors, and fibrinolytic agents.

19. The primary purpose of anticoagulants when administered after a blood clot is discovered is to: *(401)*
    1. prevent the clot from forming.
    2. dissolve the existing clot.
    3. prevent the extension of the existing clot.
    4. decrease the size of the clot.
20. When a small fragment of a thrombus breaks off and circulates until it becomes trapped causing a cerebral embolism, the treatment of choice would be to use a(n): *(417)*
    1. thrombin inhibitor.

2. anticoagulant.
3. platelet inhibitor.
4. fibrinolytic agent.

21. Platelet inhibitors are used to prevent clot formation in conditions such as: *(Select all that apply.)* *(403)*
    1. mitral stenosis.
    2. strokes (CVAs).
    3. transient ischemic attacks (TIAs).
    4. myocardial infarction.
    5. thrombocytopenia.
22. When patients are receiving anticoagulants, the nurse should instruct them on measures to prevent clot formation such as: *(Select all that apply.)* *(402)*
    1. active or passive leg exercises.
    2. not to flex the knees.
    3. placing pressure against the popliteal space behind the knees.
    4. regular ambulation.
    5. standing or sitting motionless for prolonged periods of time.
23. Which adverse effects need to be reported when patients are taking apixaban (Eliquis)? *(Select all that apply.)* *(407)*
    1. Nystagmus
    2. Easy bruising
    3. Black tarry stools
    4. Ataxia
    5. Hematuria
24. The therapeutic effect of heparin is monitored by which laboratory test? *(412)*
    1. Protime
    2. Platelets
    3. aPTT
    4. Hematocrit
25. The thrombin inhibitor dabigatran (Pradaxa) has which major advantage over anticoagulants used for reducing the risk of stroke or systemic embolism? *(416)*
    1. When metabolized, it takes the form of four active metabolites.
    2. The drug does not require monitoring of blood tests to adjust the dosage.
    3. The capsules are taken two times daily with or without food.
    4. Baseline blood pressure readings need to be obtained supine and standing.

Describe specific monitoring procedures and laboratory data used to detect hemorrhage in the patient taking anticoagulants.

26. Which premedication assessments should be performed by the nurse before administering aspirin as a platelet inhibitor? *(Select all that apply.)* *403)*
    1. Concurrent use of antihypertensives
    2. Gastrointestinal symptoms
    3. Neurologic assessment
    4. Baseline serum glucose if on oral hypoglycemic
    5. Serum potassium levels

27. The nurse will observe for which specific events to detect hemorrhage in patients on IV heparin? *(Select all that apply.)* *(414)*
    1. Decreasing blood pressure
    2. Cold, clammy skin
    3. Increasing pulse
    4. Paresthesias
    5. Disoriented sensorium
28. Nurses will educate patients on what to report when on Coumadin therapy and include which symptoms, which may indicate a need to check the INR? *(Select all that apply.)* *(415)*
    1. Tarry stools
    2. Nosebleeds
    3. Claudication
    4. Coffee-ground or blood-tinged vomitus
    5. Petechiae
29. The nurse who is preparing to start a patient on IV heparin as ordered knows that which procedures need to be done to ensure the correct dose is administered? *(Select all that apply.)* *(413-414)*
    1. Asking another nurse to check calculations and the proper heparin strength
    2. Monitoring the infusion at least every 30–60 minutes
    3. Monitor the patient for hematocrit, platelet counts, and aPTT levels
    4. Anticipate the dose will be 70–100 units/kg/hour for the infusion
    5. Assess for signs of bleeding
30. An order for subcutaneous heparin was received by the nurse, who will prepare and administer the drug after reviewing which precautions? *(Select all that apply.)* *(413)*
    1. Obtain the correct needle length—usually 1/2 inch.
    2. Avoid rotating sites of injection.
    3. Plan to use the abdominal area.
    4. After injecting the drug, massage the area for 10 seconds.
    5. Avoid an area of 2 inches around the umbilicus.
31. When administering heparin, the nurse knows that this drug can be administered by which routes? *(413)*
    1. Orally, subcutaneously, IV
    2. IM, subcutaneously, IV
    3. Orally, IM, IV
    4. Subcutaneously, IV
32. It is appropriate to give only half the dose of protamine if it is given: *(414)*
    1. less than 15 minutes after the heparin.
    2. more than 30 minutes after the heparin.
    3. less than 30 minutes after the heparin.
    4. more than 60 minutes after the heparin.

Describe the nursing assessments needed to monitor therapeutic response and adverse effects from anticoagulant therapy.

33. What therapeutic response does the nurse need to monitor when patients are on warfarin (Coumadin)? *(414)*
    1. The prothrombin time (PT) or INR results will be within the recommended range.
    2. Urine may appear red, smoke-colored, or brownish.
    3. Occult blood will be evident in stools.
    4. The skin and mucous membranes will have petechiae, ecchymosis, or hematomas.
34. Which adverse effect from warfarin (Coumadin) indicates that the patient is bleeding under the skin? *(415)*
    1. Thrombocytopenia
    2. Hematuria
    3. Petechiae
    4. Anemia
35. What measures are available for patients who have a supratherapeutic effect of warfarin (Coumadin)? *(415)*
    1. Administration of niacin (vitamin B_3)
    2. Administration of vitamin K and sometimes plasma
    3. Administration of naloxone (Narcan) as an antidote
    4. Administration of protamine sulfate as an antidote
36. What is the normal therapeutic range of International Normalized Ratio (INR) for warfarin (Coumadin) therapy for a patient with a mechanical prosthetic heart valve? *(414)*
    1. 1.5–2.0
    2. 2.0–3.0
    3. 2.5–3.5
    4. 3.0–3.5

Drugs Used to Treat Heart Failure

Answer Key: Textbook page references are provided as a guide for answering these questions. A complete answer key is provided to your instructor.

MATCHING
Match the definition on the right with the key term on the left.

	Term		Definition
1.	_____ systolic dysfunction	a.	having the ability to slow the heart rate
2.	_____ diastolic dysfunction	b.	when the heart lacks sufficient force to pump all the blood
3.	_____ inotropic agents	c.	signs and symptoms include anorexia, nausea, and bradycardia
4.	_____ digitalis toxicity	d.	when the heart fails to relax enough between contractions to allow adequate filling
5.	_____ negative chronotropy	e.	having the ability to stimulate the heart to increase the force of contractions

REVIEW QUESTIONS

Scenario: An 88-year-old male patient was admitted to the hospital with the diagnosis of exacerbation of heart failure. He has a history of coronary artery disease (CAD) with a stent placed in the past, pulmonary hypertension, hyperlipidemia, and asthma.

Explain heart failure in terms of the body's compensatory mechanisms.

6. The patient in the scenario has symptoms of systolic dysfunction of the heart causing decreased cardiac output and decreased tissue perfusion. What can the nurse expect to find upon assessment? *(Select all that apply.)* *(424)*
    1. Peripheral edema
    2. Fatigue
    3. Bradycardia
    4. Shortness of breath
    5. Exercise intolerance

7. What is the ultimate problem associated with diastolic dysfunction of the heart? *(419)*
    1. The residual blood volume remains from the previous contraction and the left ventricle does not fill adequately prior to the next contraction.
    2. The left ventricle becomes soft and boggy from being distended.
    3. The symptoms of pulmonary embolism develop.
    4. The peripheral vasculature develops stiffness.

8. When patients are in heart failure, the kidneys respond to the decreased perfusion via the renin-angiotensin-aldosterone system, which stimulates the renal distal tubules to increase blood volume by: *(420)*
    1. releasing epinephrine and norepinephrine.
    2. increasing renin production.
    3. excreting excess fluid.
    4. retaining sodium and water.

Identify the goals of treatment of heart failure.

9. The patient in the scenario has which underlying diseases that are treated to correct the heart failure? *(Select all that apply.)* *(421)*
    1. Hyperlipidemia
    2. Thyroid disease
    3. CAD
    4. Hypertension
    5. Asthma

10. The goals of treatment of heart failure include: *(Select all that apply.)* *(420)*
    1. being able to use only one drug to improve symptoms.
    2. prolongation of life.
    3. increased exercise tolerance.
    4. reduction of signs and symptoms of fluid overload.
    5. increasing intravascular volume.

11. The patient in the scenario will be educated by the nurse on which lifestyle changes that are aimed at improving heart failure? *(Select all that apply.)* *(421)*

1. Explore coping mechanisms the person uses in response to stress.
2. Discuss adaptations needed at home to find positions for relief of dyspnea.
3. Provide instructions for taking the blood pressure, pulse, and respirations.
4. Discuss spacing activities of daily living to conserve energy and avoid fatigue.
5. Provide food choices for a general diet with no fluid restrictions.

Identify the primary actions on heart failure of digoxin, angiotensin-converting enzyme inhibitors, and beta blockers.

12. What are the desired therapeutic outcomes of digitalis glycosides (digoxin) for the treatment of heart failure? *(Select all that apply.)* *(428)*
    1. Improved tolerance of activity
    2. Tolerating oxygen therapy during rest
    3. Improved cardiac output resulting in improved tissue perfusion
    4. Improvement of dyspnea
    5. Maintaining a serum digoxin level of 2.0 ng/mL
13. The angiotensin-converting enzyme (ACE) inhibitors are used primarily in heart failure because they: *(427)*
    1. increase the secretion of aldosterone.
    2. stimulate the heart to increase the force of contractions.
    3. reduce afterload by blocking vasoconstriction.
    4. increase sodium excretion.
14. The drug class of beta-adrenergic blocking agents reduces blood pressure and is also used for heart failure patients because it is thought to: *(428)*
    1. increase sodium excretion.
    2. inhibit renin release to improve symptoms of heart failure.
    3. increase the secretion of aldosterone.
    4. stimulate the renin-angiotensin-aldosterone system.

Describe digoxin toxicity and ways to prevent it.

15. The nurse will monitor which laboratory results of a patient who is on digoxin? *(Select all that apply.)* *(429)*
    1. Serum potassium
    2. Serum sodium
    3. Digoxin level
    4. Protime
    5. Serum creatinine
16. When a patient with heart failure on multiple medications is complaining of loss of appetite or any nausea or vomiting, as well as extreme fatigue, nightmares, and perhaps visual disturbances, the nurse should be alert to consider: *(429)*
    1. worsening of heart failure.
    2. digoxin toxicity.
    3. dysrhythmias.
    4. noncompliance with medications.

17. In addition to hypokalemia, other clinical conditions that may also induce digitalis toxicity include: *(Select all that apply.)* *(430)*
    1. hypertension.
    2. acute myocardial infarction.
    3. hypothyroidism.
    4. renal disease.
    5. severe respiratory disease.
18. Before initiating digoxin therapy, the nurse will obtain baseline data such as: *(Select all that apply.)* *(428)*
    1. weight.
    2. vital signs.
    3. apical pulse for one full minute.
    4. lung sounds.
    5. serum digoxin level.
19. The nurse will take an apical pulse for 1 full minute before administering digoxin, and notify the prescriber if he or she detects a pulse less than: *(428)*
    1. 60 or greater than 90 beats per minute.
    2. 40 or greater than 120 beats per minute.
    3. 60 or greater than 100 beats per minute.
    4. 75 or greater than 120 beats per minute.
20. The patient should be monitored for development of digitalis toxicity, which can be exacerbated by the presence of: *(429)*
    1. hypokalemia and hypermagnesemia.
    2. hypokalemia and hypomagnesemia.
    3. hyperkalemia and hypomagnesemia.
    4. hyperkalemia and hypermagnesemia.

Identify essential assessment data and nursing interventions needed for a patient with heart failure.

21. The nurse is teaching the patient in the scenario important health promotion measures and will emphasize the need for: *(Select all that apply.)* *(425-426)*
    1. short-term treatment.
    2. lifelong treatment.
    3. exercise regimens.
    4. proper diet.
    5. identifying signs and symptoms of worsening heart failure.
22. Which drug classes are used to treat heart failure? *(Select all that apply.)* *(421)*
    1. Fibric acids
    2. Nitrates
    3. ACE inhibitors
    4. Diuretics
    5. Hypoglycemic agents
23. The six cardinal signs of heart disease associated with inadequate tissue perfusion include: *(424)*
    1. dyspnea, edema, chest pain, syncope, fatigue, palpitations.
    2. hypotension, dyspnea, chest pain, tachycardia, lightheadedness, hypokalemia.
    3. syncope, palpitations, tachycardia, atrial fibrillation, chest pain, edema.
    4. palpitations, atrial fibrillation, chest pain, syncope, edema, bradycardia.

Drugs Used for Diuresis

Answer Key: Textbook page references are provided as a guide for answering these questions. A complete answer key is provided to your instructor.

MATCHING

Match the drug class on the right with the drug name on the left. Drug class options can be used more than once.

Drug Name	Drug Class
1. _____ chlorothiazide	a. sulfonamide-type loop diuretics
2. _____ acetazolamide	b. carbonic anhydrase inhibitor
3. _____ furosemide	c. thiazide diuretics
4. _____ triamterene	d. potassium-sparing diuretics
5. _____ spironolactone	
6. _____ bumetanide	

REVIEW QUESTIONS

Scenario: A 74-year-old male patient was admitted to the hospital with a recent urinary tract infection. It was subsequently found that the patient had hyponatremia, with an acute kidney injury and history of hypertension and heart failure.

Identify the nursing assessments used to evaluate a patient's state of hydration and renal function.

7. When assessing a patient who is overhydrated, which assessment finding does the nurse expect to see? *(433)*
   1. Poor skin turgor
   2. Deteriorating vital signs
   3. Deeply furrowed tongue
   4. Neck vein engorgement
8. What are the classic signs of dehydration that the nurse will assess for and report? *(Select all that apply.)* *(433)*
   1. Shrunken or deeply furrowed tongue
   2. Skin turgor elastic with rapid return to flat position
   3. Delayed capillary filling
   4. Soft or sunken eyeballs
   5. Weak pedal pulses
9. A patient who has received IV fluids in excess of fluids excreted is likely to develop which signs? *(Select all that apply.)* *(433)*
   1. Peripheral edema
   2. Presence of crackles
   3. Sunken eyeballs
   4. Hypernatremia
   5. Muscle cramps
10. When taking a history of a patient with fluid volume excess, the nurse should ask the patient questions relating to any history of heart disorders that contribute to fluid volume excess such as: *(Select all that apply.)* *(433)*
    1. endocarditis.
    2. dysrhythmias.
    3. heart failure.
    4. myocardial infarction.
    5. patent foramen ovale (PFO).
11. Patients with which conditions are prone to developing fluid volume excess? *(Select all that apply.)* *(433)*
    1. Hypertension
    2. Heart failure
    3. Renal disease (renal failure)
    4. Hypothyroidism
    5. Ascites
12. The nurse should be aware of factors that may predispose a patient to the development of fluid volume excess such as: *(Select all that apply.)* *(433)*
    1. immobility.
    2. diuretic agents.
    3. corticosteroid agents.
    4. hypertension.
    5. pregnancy.

13. What laboratory tests should the nurse monitor to determine if the patient has impaired kidney function? *(433)*
    1. Potassium and sodium
    2. BUN and serum creatinine
    3. Hemoglobin and hematocrit
    4. Platelets and protime
14. What laboratory studies should be performed whenever a diuretic is prescribed? *(Select all that apply.)* *(433)*
    1. Potassium
    2. Hematocrit
    3. Sodium
    4. BUN and creatinine
    5. Platelets
15. The nurse will assess which laboratory results for the patient in the scenario to determine the extent of kidney injury? *(433)*
    1. Potassium and sodium
    2. WBC
    3. BUN and creatinine
    4. Hemoglobin and hematocrit

Describe the actions of diuretics and their effects on blood pressure and electrolytes.

16. The therapeutic outcomes associated with diuretic therapy include: *(Select all that apply.)* *(436)*
    1. decreased potassium level.
    2. improvement in the symptoms of fluid volume excess.
    3. reduced edema.
    4. reduced blood pressure.
    5. decreasing the excretory load on the kidneys.
17. The patient in the scenario is currently taking digoxin (Lanoxin), aminoglycosides, nonsteroidal antiinflammatory drugs (NSAIDs), and corticosteroids for multiple medical problems. Which principle does the nurse consider in monitoring this patient when bumetanide (Bumex) has now been prescribed? *(437)*
    1. The amount of digoxin will need to be increased.
    2. The potential for ototoxicity from the aminoglycosides is increased.
    3. The dose of bumetanide will need to be decreased when also taking NSAIDs.
    4. The use of corticosteroids and bumetanide may cause hyperkalemia.
18. A patient with type 2 diabetes mellitus and congestive heart failure is being treated with metformin (Glucophage), warfarin (Coumadin), and digitalis. The patient has a new order for bumetanide (Bumex). What adverse effects does the nurse watch for? *(Select all that apply.)* *(437)*
    1. Orthostatic hypotension
    2. Fluid overload
    3. Dry mouth
    4. Edema
    5. Electrolyte imbalance

19. The patient who has experienced vomiting and diarrhea is likely to develop which type of electrolyte imbalance? *(434)*
    1. Hypomagnesemia
    2. Hypernatremia
    3. Hyperkalemia
    4. Hypokalemia
20. When monitoring the laboratory values of potassium in patients taking diuretics, the nurse knows the normal value for potassium is: *(434)*
    1. 135 mEq/L to 147 mEq/L.
    2. 3.5 mEq/L to 5.5 mEq/L.
    3. 1.6 mEq/L to 2.4 mEq/L.
    4. 2.5 mg/dL to 4.5 mg/dL.
21. Thiazides may cause or aggravate an imbalance in which electrolyte? *(Select all that apply.)* *(440)*
    1. Chloride (Cl^-)
    2. Potassium (K^+)
    3. Sodium (Na^+)
    4. Magnesium (Mg^+)
    5. Calcium (Ca^+)
22. When thiazide diuretics such as chlorothiazide (Diuril) are administered, the drug is acting primarily on the: *(439)*
    1. enzyme in the kidneys that promotes excretion of sodium and water.
    2. ascending limb of the loop of Henle.
    3. distal tubules of the kidneys.
    4. descending limb of the loop of Henle.
23. Carbonic anhydrase inhibitors are used as a mild diuretic, and also as an effective agent for: *(436)*
    1. hypothyroidism.
    2. glaucoma.
    3. gouty arthritis.
    4. peripheral neuropathy.
24. Potent diuretics that act primarily by inhibiting sodium and chloride reabsorption from the ascending limb of the loop of Henle in the kidneys include: *(Select all that apply.)* *(436)*
    1. bumetanide.
    2. metolazone.
    3. furosemide.
    4. acetazolamide.
    5. torsemide.

Explain the rationale for administering diuretics cautiously to older adults and individuals with impaired renal function, cirrhosis of the liver, or diabetes mellitus.

25. The patient in the scenario has the diagnosis of hyponatremia, which in this case is caused by: *(Select all that apply.)* *(433-434)*
    1. urinary tract infection.
    2. heart failure.
    3. fluid overload secondary to kidney impairment.
    4. hypertension.
    5. diabetes.

26. When administering thiazide and loop diuretics to a diabetic patient, the nurse will need to monitor what lab results to prevent an adverse reaction? *(Select all that apply.)* *(438)*
    1. Potassium
    2. Blood sugar
    3. Sodium
    4. Hemoglobin
    5. Prothrombin time
27. A patient taking ethacrynic acid (Edecrin) is most at risk for developing dizziness, deafness, and tinnitus when he or she also has which condition? *(438)*
    1. Liver disease
    2. A hearing deficit
    3. Impaired renal function
    4. History of myocardial infarction
28. The patient with glaucoma who is receiving acetazolamide (Diamox) can expect which effect? *(435)*
    1. Increased urine output
    2. Rapid heart rate
    3. Nasal congestion
    4. Insomnia
29. The nurse discussed with the patient in the scenario which reasons for the medication furosemide (Lasix) that was prescribed? *(Select all that apply.)* *(436)*
    1. "The Lasix will help you get rid of excess fluid that your heart failure is causing."
    2. "We are using the Lasix to treat your urinary tract infection."
    3. "Lasix is the drug we give patients who have hypotension."
    4. "Your hypertension and heart failure can be improved with the use of Lasix."
    5. "This drug will induce hypernatremia to treat your hyponatremia."
30. Diuretic therapy has been shown to be effective in reducing edema and improving symptoms of: *(432)*
    1. hyperuricemia.
    2. hyperglycemia.
    3. heart failure.
    4. hypokalemia.
31. Which statements does the nurse include when teaching a patient about diuretic therapy? *(Select all that apply.)* *(435)*
    1. "If you are taking Aldactone, avoid the use of salt substitutes in your diet."
    2. "You should rise slowly from a lying or sitting position and lie down if you feel faint, because some diuretics cause you to develop low blood pressure in certain positions."
    3. "You should take your diuretic pill before you go to sleep."
    4. "Weigh yourself every day and call your primary healthcare provider if you note a 1-lb weight gain in 1 day."
    5. "The purpose of diuretics is to increase the net loss of water."

32. The nurse gives which instructions to a patient who is on hydrochlorothiazide (HydroDIURIL) on how to reduce indigestion that the patient is experiencing? *(439)*
    1. "This medication will cause gastric irritation no matter what you do."
    2. "Take this medication with food or milk to reduce gastric irritation."
    3. "Always take this medication on an empty stomach."
    4. "It is best to take this medication with at least 8 oz of water."
33. If patients take salt substitutes while on spironolactone (Aldactone), the patient's laboratory results may indicate: *(442)*
    1. hypokalemia.
    2. hyponatremia.
    3. hypercalcemia.
    4. hyperkalemia.

Identify the nursing assessments needed to monitor the therapeutic response or the development of common or serious adverse effects of diuretic therapy.

34. What patient assessments should be performed on a regular basis when diuretics are being administered? *(Select all that apply.)* *(434)*
    1. Presence of edema
    2. Intake and output
    3. Blood pressure
    4. Activity intolerance
    5. Daily weights
35. The nurse observes the patient for signs of adverse effects from diuretic therapy mainly from electrolyte imbalance, which will be in the form of: *(Select all that apply.)* *(437)*
    1. tremors.
    2. muscle cramps.
    3. nocturia.
    4. nausea.
    5. altered mental status.
36. A male patient with hypertension is prescribed spironolactone (Aldactone) therapy. Which instruction does the nurse include when teaching the patient about this therapy? *(442)*
    1. "Avoid salt in your diet as well as salt substitutes."
    2. "Take spironolactone on an empty stomach."
    3. "Be sure to increase the amounts of tomatoes and citrus in your diet."
    4. "If you develop breast tenderness, immediately stop taking the spironolactone."

Drugs Used to Treat Upper Respiratory Disease

chapter
29

Answer Key: Textbook page references are provided as a guide for answering these questions. A complete answer key is provided to your instructor.

MATCHING

Match the drug class on the right with the drug name on the left. Drug class options can be used more than once.

Drug Name

1. _____ cetirizine
2. _____ desloratadine
3. _____ loratadine
4. _____ naphazoline
5. _____ oxymetazoline
6. _____ triamcinolone
7. _____ xylometazoline

Drug Class

a. nasal decongestants
b. antihistamines
c. intranasal corticosteroids

REVIEW QUESTIONS

Scenario: A 48-year-old male patient came into the clinic complaining of itchy, red eyes and frequent sneezing with nasal congestion. He was diagnosed with allergic rhinitis.

Describe the function of the respiratory system and list the common upper respiratory diseases.

8. The respiratory function of the nose is to do what to the inhaled air prior to its traveling into the lower respiratory airways? *(Select all that apply.) (446)*
   1. Detect odors
   2. Humidify
   3. React to allergens by sneezing
   4. Warm
   5. Filter
9. The upper respiratory tract is composed of which structures? *(Select all that apply.) (446)*
   1. Eustachian tubes
   2. Tonsils
   3. Turbinates
   4. Pharynx
   5. Lacrimal ducts
10. Which upper respiratory condition is actually a bacterial infection? *(448)*
    1. Sinusitis
    2. Common cold

3. Allergic rhinitis
4. Rhinitis medicamentosa

Discuss the causes of allergic rhinitis and nasal congestion and rhinitis medicamentosa.

11. What response does histamine release cause in the mucous membranes of the nose? *(448)*
    1. Stimulation of the olfactory cells
    2. Increased surface area of the nasal passages
    3. Decreased ciliary movement
    4. Urticaria, redness, and edema
12. The patient's symptoms in the scenario were probably caused by exposure to which allergens? *(Select all that apply.) (448)*
    1. Dust mites
    2. Viruses
    3. Pollens
    4. Animal dander
    5. Grasses
13. Which findings does the nurse typically assess in a patient experiencing a severe allergic reaction? *(Select all that apply.) (448)*
    1. Hypertension
    2. Dry skin
    3. Urticaria
    4. Bronchospasms
    5. Tachycardia

14. When patients overuse topical decongestants, this can lead to rebound secretions caused by excessive vasoconstriction of the blood vessels in the nasal membranes called: *(448)*
    1. allergic rhinitis.
    2. rhinorrhea.
    3. rhinitis medicamentosa.
    4. sinusitis.
15. The nurse educating a patient on ways to treat rhinitis medicamentosa should provide the patient which instructions? *(Select all that apply.)* *(449)*
    1. "The best treatment for this condition is to avoid it in the first place."
    2. "There are several treatment options available for you, but first it is important to understand the cause of the problem."
    3. "One option for you would be to completely stop taking the decongestant and work through the discomfort you will experience."
    4. "One option for you would be to work to clear one nostril at a time."
    5. "One option for you would be to switch to another decongestant—one that will not cause this condition."
16. A patient in the scenario was asking the nurse what would be recommended to treat his nasal congestion from allergy symptoms. The best response from the nurse would be: *(448)*
    1. "You should avoid topical decongestants as their use could cause a rebound problem that is difficult to treat."
    2. "It does not matter what type of decongestant you use, they are all very similar."
    3. "Only use prescription medications, as the over-the-counter medications often do not work for people."
    4. "To eliminate your symptoms, you simply must avoid the allergen."

Explain the major actions (effects) of sympathomimetic, antihistaminic, and corticosteroid decongestants and cromolyn.

17. The potential anticholinergic adverse effects of antihistamine therapy include: *(Select all that apply.)* *(452)*
    1. diarrhea.
    2. blurred vision.
    3. dry mouth.
    4. urinary retention.
    5. stuffy nose.
18. Antihistamines such as fexofenadine (Allegra) are H_1 receptor antagonists and they work by: *(452)*
    1. eliciting the production of a specific antibody against an allergen.
    2. constricting the blood vessels in the nasal passages.
    3. blocking the H_1 receptor sites on the target cells.
    4. causing sedation and dryness of mucous membranes.

19. What occurs when patients with allergic seasonal rhinitis do not respond to antihistamines? *(Select all that apply.)* *(452)*
    1. Nasal itching
    2. Sneezing
    3. Rhinorrhea
    4. Nasal congestion
    5. Lacrimation
20. Which statement does the nurse include when teaching a patient about the use of cromolyn sodium (Nasalcrom)? *(456)*
    1. "Cromolyn sodium should be administered after the body receives a stimulus to release histamine."
    2. "Cromolyn sodium causes bronchodilation."
    3. "A 2- to 4-week course of therapy is usually required to determine clinical response."
    4. "Cromolyn sodium should be discontinued when the desired therapeutic response is achieved."

Explain why all decongestant products should be used cautiously by people with hypertension, hyperthyroidism, diabetes mellitus, cardiac disease, increased intraocular pressure, or prostatic disease.

21. The nurse consults the prescriber before administering a sympathomimetic decongestant to patients with which conditions? *(Select all that apply.)* *(451)*
    1. Diabetes mellitus
    2. Glaucoma
    3. Allergy to shellfish
    4. Hypothyroidism
    5. Prostatic hyperplasia
22. When patients use nasal decongestants such as pseudoephedrine, they must be aware of the possible resulting hypertension, because the sympathomimetic decongestants' action is one of: *(450)*
    1. vasodilation.
    2. vasoconstriction.
    3. bronchoconstriction.
    4. bronchodilation.
23. The patient in the scenario also has hyperthyroidism, which prompted the nurse to caution the patient regarding the use of sympathomimetic decongestants because these agents will: *(451)*
    1. cause eye irritation and lacrimation.
    2. produce stinging to the nasal membranes.
    3. have no effect on allergic rhinitis.
    4. stimulate alpha receptors.

Discuss the premedication assessments and nursing assessments needed during therapy to monitor the therapeutic response to and the common and serious adverse effects of decongestant drug therapy.

24. When a drug monograph says that a drug produces anticholinergic effects, the nurse anticipates that which symptoms may occur? *(Select all that apply.)* *(452)*

1. Nasal congestion
2. Constipation
3. Urinary retention
4. Dry mouth
5. Blurred vision

25. The nurse recognizes that which adverse effects can be anticipated whenever an antihistamine is administered? *(454)*
    1. Rhinorrhea and lacrimation
    2. Urticaria and blurred vision
    3. Sedation and dry mouth
    4. Urinary retention and constipation

26. What is the paradoxical effect from antihistamines often seen in children and older adults? *(449)*
    1. Insomnia, nervousness, and irritability
    2. Sedation and lethargy
    3. Sneezing and rhinorrhea
    4. Nasal congestion and pruritus

27. What important patient education instructions will the nurse include for patients who will be started on antihistamines? *(Select all that apply.)* *(454)*
    1. Exercise caution when operating any power equipment or while driving because of the medication's sedative effects.
    2. Maintain adequate hydration.
    3. Take a dose immediately upon recognition of an allergic response (for unanticipated exposure).

4. Take the dose 30–45 minutes prior to possible exposure to block receptors.
5. Expect relief from runny nose and eyes, itching, and nasal congestion.

28. When teaching adult patients with blocked nasal passages about the correct order to administer their medications, the nurse will instruct them to: *(456)*
    1. administer their intranasal corticosteroid before any decongestant.
    2. administer a nasal decongestant just before the intranasal cromolyn sodium (Nasalcrom).
    3. administer their antihistamine 30 minutes prior to the use of any decongestants.
    4. avoid using a nasal decongestant; use their intranasal corticosteroid instead.

29. Which statements about cromolyn sodium (Nasalcrom) are true? *(Select all that apply.)* *(456)*
    1. Cromolyn must be taken before exposure to the stimulus that initiates an attack of allergic rhinitis.
    2. Cromolyn has no direct bronchodilation or antihistamine effects.
    3. Cromolyn does not relieve nasal congestion.
    4. Patients who experience coughing when taking cromolyn should notify their primary healthcare provider.
    5. The full therapeutic benefit is usually not evident until after 3 to 6 weeks of therapy.

Drugs Used to Treat Lower Respiratory Disease

chapter

30

Answer Key: Textbook page references are provided as a guide for answering these questions. A complete answer key is provided to your instructor.

MATCHING

Match the definition on the right with the key term on the left.

Key Term

1. _____ ventilation
2. _____ diffusion
3. _____ asthma
4. _____ bronchospasm
5. _____ goblet cells
6. _____ bronchitis

Definition

a. the movement of air in and out of the lungs
b. smooth muscle constriction causing narrowing of the airways
c. specialized mucous glands of the respiratory tract
d. a common inflammatory disease of the bronchi and bronchioles
e. a condition causing inflammation and edema with excessive mucus secretion
f. the process by which oxygen passes across the alveolar membrane to the blood

REVIEW QUESTIONS

Scenario: A 75-year-old male patient was admitted to the hospital with respiratory failure secondary to pneumonia. After several days of being treated with steroids and antibiotics, he has stabilized on 2 liters of oxygen via nasal cannula. He has a history of chronic obstructive pulmonary disease (COPD), congestive heart failure, hypothyroidism, and rheumatoid arthritis, all of which are currently medically managed.

Compare the physiologic responses of the respiratory system to emphysema, chronic bronchitis, and asthma.

7. Which airway disease is characterized by restricted alveolar expansion due to loss of elasticity of tissue or physical deformity of the chest itself? *(460)*
   1. Reactive airway disease
   2. Obstructive airway disease
   3. Restrictive airway disease
   4. Resistive airway disease
8. Asthma is best described as a(n): *(461)*
   1. inflammatory disease of the bronchi and bronchioles.
   2. restrictive airway disease of the trachea.
   3. constrictive disease of the bronchi and bronchioles.
   4. perfusion/ventilation disproportion condition.
9. Obstructive airway diseases, which are caused by narrowing of the airway, occur when which conditions are present? *(Select all that apply.) (459-460)*
   1. Edema
   2. Bronchospasm
   3. Decreased perfusion
   4. Inflammation of the bronchial walls
   5. Excess mucus secretion
10. Examples of obstructive lung diseases in which the airway passages are narrowed and increased resistance to airflow occurs are: *(Select all that apply.) (460)*
    1. pulmonary fibrosis.
    2. asthma.
    3. emphysema.
    4. acute bronchitis.
    5. kyphoscoliosis.
11. What is the process by which oxygen passes across the alveolar membrane to the blood in the capillaries? *(459)*
    1. Ventilation
    2. Diffusion
    3. Perfusion
    4. Osmosis
12. The respiratory tract normally produces thin, watery secretions to form a thin layer of fluid over the interior surfaces of the respiratory tract. This fluid originates from: *(459)*
    1. cilia and alveolar membranes.
    2. mucous glands and serous glands.
    3. sebaceous glands and nasal mucosa.
    4. goblet cells and mast cells.
13. The important components of blood gases that nurses need to monitor that indicate overall pulmonary function are: *(Select all that apply.) (460)*

1. Pao$_2$.
2. pH.
3. Paco$_2$.
4. HCO$_3$.
5. Hgb.
14. Which component of blood gases measures the ratio of actual oxygen content of hemoglobin compared with the hemoglobin's ability to carry oxygen? *(460)*
    1. Sao$_2$
    2. Pao$_2$
    3. pH
    4. Paco$_2$

Cite nursing assessments used to evaluate the respiratory status of a patient.

15. A nurse is assessing the patient in the scenario and listens to lung sounds. Which findings would the nurse report to the healthcare provider for further evaluation? *(460, 466)*
    1. Coarse crackles throughout lung fields
    2. Diminished breath sounds at the bases
    3. Coughing up thick, yellow secretions
    4. Rapid, shallow breathing with O$_2$ saturation of 88%
16. During a respiratory assessment of the patient in the scenario, the nurse listens to breath sounds and monitors the respiratory rate, as well as: *(Select all that apply.) (466)*
    1. use of abdominal muscles during breathing.
    2. appetite.
    3. mental status.
    4. signs of cyanosis.
    5. pulse rate.
17. Laboratory and diagnostic tests are also checked as part of the respiratory assessment that the nurse monitors, including: *(Select all that apply.) (466)*
    1. pulmonary function tests.
    2. creatinine clearance.
    3. electrocardiograph.
    4. ABGs.
    5. chest x-rays.
18. The nurse needs to educate patients who have respiratory conditions on important health maintenance aspects such as: *(Select all that apply.) (467)*
    1. dietary and hydration needs.
    2. balancing activities with abilities.
    3. environmental control with filtration systems.
    4. use of abdominal muscles during breathing.
    5. pulmonary hygiene.
19. The nurse was discussing the timing of the administration of medications for a patient with asthma. Which statement by the nurse is correct? *(467)*
    1. "It does not matter in which order you take your medications."
    2. "Take your steroid inhaler first, then your bronchodilator."
    3. "Take your bronchodilator first, then your steroid inhaler."

4. "Take your bronchodilator first, then wait 2 hours before taking your steroid inhaler."
20. The nurse is explaining the different zones of a peak flowmeter to the patient with asthma and how to use it to assess when her symptoms are changing. The nurse recognizes that the patient needs further teaching after she states: *(467)*
    1. "The green zone is good, the yellow zone is warning, and the red zone is danger."
    2. "I can use the quick-relief medication when I notice that I am in the yellow zone."
    3. "The quick-relief medication and corticosteroids are used when I am in the green zone."
    4. "The peak flowmeter measures my peak expiratory flow and helps me determine how to manage my asthma."

Distinguish the mechanisms of action of expectorants, antitussives, and mucolytic agents.

21. Which drug is an effective cough suppressant and the standard against which other antitussive agents are compared? *(470)*
    1. Dextromethorphan (Delsym)
    2. Acetylcysteine (Mucomyst)
    3. Guaifenesin (Robitussin)
    4. Codeine
22. Expectorants are those drugs whose action is to: *(469)*
    1. enhance the flow of respiratory secretions, which promotes ciliary action.
    2. increase the viscosity of mucus plugs.
    3. suppress the cough center in the brain.
    4. relax the smooth muscles of the airway.
23. The nurse was educating the patient on what to expect from mucolytics, and described them as: *(470)*
    1. agents that play an important role in the treatment of asthma to reduce inflammation.
    2. agents that reduce the stickiness and viscosity of pulmonary secretions by acting directly on the mucus plugs to dissolve them.
    3. agents that relax the smooth muscle of the tracheobronchial tree.
    4. agents that may produce a goiter when used over an extended length of time in children.
24. The nurse gives a patient which instructions prior to the administration of an antitussive agent? *(Select all that apply.) (470)*
    1. Ensure nebulizing equipment is available for administration.
    2. Caution the patient regarding sedative effects.
    3. Describe the characteristics of the cough.
    4. Record peak expiratory flow prior to use.
    5. Ensure the patient keeps well-hydrated.
25. When administering guaifenesin (Robitussin) to a patient with bronchitis, the nurse expects that the drug will: *(469)*
    1. increase the frequency of a nonproductive cough.
    2. dilate the bronchioles.

3. increase the viscosity of mucus secretions.
4. thin the bronchial secretions.
26. The nurse will assess the action of acetylcysteine as working when the patient exhibits: *(471)*
    1. increased nonproductive coughing.
    2. improved airway flow and more comfortable breathing.
    3. thicker and more viscous secretions.
    4. Kussmaul's respirations.

Describe the nursing assessments needed to monitor therapeutic response and the development of adverse effects from beta-adrenergic bronchodilator therapy.

27. What actions do beta-adrenergic agents have on patients with respiratory conditions such as asthma? *(472)*
    1. Bronchodilation
    2. Decrease in peak expiratory flow
    3. Thinner respiratory secretions
    4. Increase in respiratory rate
28. The patient in the scenario was given beta-adrenergic agents, and the nurse needs to monitor for which systemic adverse effects? *(Select all that apply.)* *(472-473)*
    1. GI disturbances
    2. Hypertension, tachycardia
    3. Insomnia, nervousness, anxiety
    4. Bradycardia, arrhythmias
    5. Sedation, lethargy
29. Short-acting beta-adrenergic agents that have a rapid onset and are used to treat acute bronchospasms include: *(Select all that apply.)* *(472)*
    1. metaproterenol.
    2. formoterol.
    3. salmeterol.
    4. albuterol.
    5. pirbuterol.

Discuss the nursing assessments needed to monitor therapeutic response and the development of adverse effects from anticholinergic bronchodilator therapy.

30. What actions do anticholinergic bronchodilator agents have on patients with respiratory conditions such as asthma? *(474)*
    1. They stabilize the mast cells to prevent the release of histamine.
    2. They block the cholinergic effect of bronchial constriction by the vagus nerve.
    3. They inhibit the inflammatory response in the bronchioles.
    4. They bind to the circulating antibodies in the blood, making them not as available to trigger symptoms.
31. What adverse effects from potent anticholinergic agents limit their use? *(Select all that apply.)* *(474)*
    1. Tachycardia

2. Urinary retention
3. Throat irritation
4. Bradycardia
5. Mydriasis

32. The following medications were ordered for the patient in the scenario. Which ones are used to treat COPD? *(Select all that apply.)* *(475, 476)*
    1. Tiotropium bromide (Spiriva)
    2. Spironolactone (Aldactone)
    3. Levothyroxine (Synthroid)
    4. Indomethacin (Indocin)
    5. Budesonide (Pulmicort)

List the lower respiratory conditions that use anticholinergic bronchodilators and corticosteroid inhalant therapy.

33. Which drugs enhance the effect of beta-adrenergic bronchodilators and inhibit inflammatory responses that may result in bronchoconstriction? *(476)*
    1. Anticholinergic bronchodilators
    2. Antileukotriene agents
    3. Corticosteroid inhalants
    4. Xanthine derivatives
34. Respiratory conditions that may be treated with any drug class—anticholinergic bronchodilators and corticosteroid inhalants—include: *(Select all that apply.)* *(474, 476)*
    1. pneumonia.
    2. bronchitis.
    3. asthma.
    4. COPD.
    5. emphysema.
35. Which patient condition is most likely to cause complications associated with beta-adrenergic bronchodilator therapy? *(472)*
    1. Diabetes mellitus
    2. Asthma
    3. Pneumonia
    4. Allergy to eggs
36. What instructions will the nurse give the patient who is started on systemic steroids for exacerbation of asthma? *(476)*
    1. "These steroids are given to allow easier breathing with less effort by decreasing bronchospasms."
    2. "Your bronchodilator inhalant agents will be discontinued while you take these steroids orally."
    3. "Your corticosteroid inhalant therapy will be discontinued while you take these steroids orally."
    4. "The full therapeutic benefit from these systemic steroids may require up to 4 weeks of therapy for maximum benefit."

Drugs Used to Treat Oral Disorders

Answer Key: Textbook page references are provided as a guide for answering these questions. A complete answer key is provided to your instructor.

MATCHING
Match the definition on the right with the key term on the left.

	Key Term		Definition
1. ____	canker sores	a.	a painful inflammation of the mucous membranes of the mouth
2. ____	candidiasis	b.	an oral fungal infection
3. ____	plaque	c.	a condition in which the flow of saliva is decreased or completely stopped
4. ____	gingivitis	d.	oral lesions usually gray to whitish yellow with a red halo of inflamed tissue
5. ____	halitosis	e.	a whitish yellow substance that builds up on teeth and gum lines
6. ____	xerostomia	f.	foul mouth odor
7. ____	mucositis	g.	inflammation of the gums

REVIEW QUESTIONS

Scenario: A 52-year-old female patient arrives at the outpatient clinic with complaints of painful mouth lesions around her lower gums. The patient was diagnosed with canker sores and treatment was started to control the pain and facilitate healing.

Explain common oral disorders and their treatments.

8. The patient in the scenario asks the nurse in the clinic what could have been done to prevent these painful sores from developing. The nurse responds: *(485)*
   1. "Everybody gets them, they will go away eventually; I would not worry about it."
   2. "Proper oral hygiene, such as brushing your teeth after eating, will prevent them."
   3. "You probably should have seen a dentist twice a year to prevent them."
   4. "The exact cause is unknown, but stress and trauma are precipitating factors."
9. The nurse was discussing with the patient who had xerostomia on the use of: *(486)*
   1. mouthwashes to freshen the breath.
   2. a saliva substitute for the condition.
   3. topical analgesics to reduce the pain.
   4. oral irrigation and proper oral hygiene.

10. Which situation can put patients at risk for the development of xerostomia? *(486)*
    1. Eating a meal with a lot of garlic
    2. Taking oral analgesics
    3. Rinsing with saline
    4. Smoking and mouth-breathing
11. Which mouth disorder is common in infants, pregnant women, and debilitated patients and is characterized by white, curd-like plaques attached to the oral mucosa? *(485)*
    1. Gingivitis
    2. Candidiasis
    3. Mucositis
    4. Xerostomia

Describe therapy used for oral health.

12. The patient in the scenario asks the nurse what she can do to minimize the pain. The nurse responds: *(Select all that apply.) (486)*
    1. "You should avoid eating foods that irritate your sores such as sharp-edged or spicy foods."
    2. "You could use a straw when drinking acidic juices or soft drinks."
    3. "Rinsing with saline may be soothing and can be done before you apply the medication."
    4. "You can use any over-the-counter mouthwash to prevent halitosis."

5. "If you apply the topical pain-relieving medication before eating or brushing your teeth, it may decrease the pain caused by these activities."

13. Patients who are being treated for cold sores should be taught by the nurse to: *(Select all that apply.)* **(486)**
    1. gently wash the cold sore with soap and water.
    2. use highly astringent products on the sores.
    3. allow the cold sore to dry so cracking can occur.
    4. keep moist to prevent drying.
    5. use saline rinses.

14. When discussing ways to prevent or treat halitosis, the nurse explains to a patient which measures to take? *(Select all that apply.)* **(487)**
    1. Brushing at least twice a day
    2. Flossing regularly
    3. Using mouthwashes
    4. Applying Vaseline to the lips
    5. Taking antifungal medications

15. Proper oral hygiene of brushing twice a day should be taught to patients to prevent what disorder? **(487)**
    1. Dental caries
    2. Canker sores
    3. Xerostomia
    4. Sinusitis

Identify nursing assessments and interventions associated with the treatment of mucositis.

16. Nurses need to perform an oral assessment in patients susceptible to mouth disorders to detect any abnormal findings such as: *(Select all that apply.)* **(488)**
    1. pink, moist mucous membranes.
    2. white patches over the tongue.

3. red, swollen gum line.
4. well-fitting dentures.
5. teeth coated with food particles.

17. Which action is most effective in providing a patient with relief of symptoms caused by mucositis? **(488)**
    1. Applying amlexanox (Aphthasol) before meals
    2. Using commercially prepared mouthwash with alcohol
    3. Avoiding exposure to the sun
    4. Using 1 tablespoon of salt or hydrogen peroxide or 1/2 teaspoon of baking soda in 8 oz of water as a mouthwash

18. A patient has severe grade 3 mucositis as determined by the World Health Organization Oral Mucositis Scale. Which medications may be ordered for the patient to treat oral mucositis? *(Select all that apply.)* **(487)**
    1. Recombinant human keratinocyte growth factor (Kepivance)
    2. Milk of Magnesia
    3. Sucralfate suspension
    4. Viscous lidocaine 2%
    5. Docosanol (Abreva)

19. When mucositis occurs after a patient receives chemotherapy, it often takes: **(487)**
    1. 5-7 days.
    2. 8-10 days.
    3. 12-14 days.
    4. 18-20 days.

Drugs Used to Treat Gastroesophageal Reflux and Peptic Ulcer Diseases

chapter
32

Answer Key: Textbook page references are provided as a guide for answering these questions. A complete answer key is provided to your instructor.

MATCHING

Match the definition on the right with the key term on the left.

Key Term

1. _____ gastroesophageal reflux disease (GERD)

2. _____ peptic ulcer disease (PUD)

3. _____ *Helicobacter pylori*

4. _____ heartburn

5. _____ mucus cells

6. _____ parietal cells

7. _____ chief cells

8. _____ hydrochloric acid

Definition

a. secretory cells of the stomach that secrete hydrochloric acid
b. acid indigestion
c. secretory cells of the stomach that secrete pepsinogen
d. symptoms include epigastric pain noted when the stomach is empty
e. bacteria that are able to live below the mucus barrier of the stomach
f. the reflux of gastric secretions up into the esophagus
g. activates pepsinogen to pepsin providing the optimal pH
h. secretory cells of the stomach that secrete mucus

REVIEW QUESTIONS

Scenario: A 38-year-old male patient came into the clinic with complaints of acid indigestion and reflux and was diagnosed with GERD and prescribed an H_2 antagonist and an antacid.

Describe the physiology of the stomach.

9. What are the major functions of the stomach? *(Select all that apply.)* **(492)**
   1. Storing food
   2. Mixing food
   3. Emptying food into the small intestine
   4. Absorbing nutrients
   5. Maintaining a pH of 6

10. Which secretory cells line the stomach and secrete pepsinogen? **(492)**
    1. Parietal cells
    2. Chief cells
    3. Mucus cells
    4. Goblet cells

11. What are the ways that the parietal cells are stimulated to produce hydrochloric acid in the stomach? *(Select all that apply.)* **(492)**
    1. By the presence of gastrin
    2. By the presence of saliva

3. By the presence of histamine
4. By acetylcholine stimulating cholinergic nerve fibers
5. By gastric amylase

Cite common stomach disorders that require drug therapy.

12. The patient in the scenario was given appropriate treatment for his GERD, but he could also have been prescribed which classes of agents? *(Select all that apply.)*? **(494)**
    1. Coating agents
    2. Proton pump inhibitors
    3. Prokinetic agents
    4. Gastrointestinal prostaglandins
    5. Antispasmodic agents

13. Which of these stomach disorders are treated with proton pump inhibitors? *(Select all that apply.)* **(500)**
    1. Gastric and duodenal ulcers
    2. Severe esophagitis
    3. GERD
    4. *Helicobacter pylori*
    5. Pyloric stenosis

14. Patients with which conditions are often placed on antispasmodic agents such as mepenzolate (Cantil) or dicyclomine (Bentyl)? *(Select all that apply.)* **(504)**

1. Esophagitis
2. Irritable bowel syndrome
3. Diverticulitis
4. Peptic ulcer disease
5. Pyloric stenosis

Identify factors that prevent breakdown of the body's normal defense barriers resulting in ulcer formation.

15. One of the known causes of peptic ulcer disease is an infection in the mucosal wall of the stomach caused by: *(493)*
    1. *Streptococcus viridans.*
    2. *Staphylococcus aureus.*
    3. *Escherichia coli.*
    4. *Helicobacter pylori.*
16. Patients older than 65 years with ulcer disease usually present with which symptoms? *(Select all that apply.)* *(496)*
    1. Weight gain
    2. Anorexia
    3. Vague abdominal discomfort
    4. Dizziness
    5. Burning in the epigastric region
17. What are the conditions that cause a breakdown in the body's defenses against ulcer disease? *(Select all that apply.)* *(493)*
    1. Excessive parietal cells secreting too much HCl
    2. Injury to the mucosal lining of the stomach by NSAIDs
    3. Stressful situations
    4. An infection in the stomach lining
    5. Spicy foods and alcohol

Discuss the drug classifications and actions used to treat stomach disorders.

18. Which class of medications is used in the treatment of peptic ulcer disease because it will block the formation of hydrochloric acid, resulting in the reduction of irritation to the gastric mucosa? *(500)*
    1. Antispasmodics
    2. Proton pump inhibitors
    3. Antacids
    4. Histamine receptor antagonists
19. Which drug is a gastric stimulant that works by increasing stomach contractions, relaxing the pyloric valve, and increasing peristalsis, as well as working as an antiemetic? *(502)*
    1. Lansoprazole (Prevacid)
    2. Ranitidine (Zantac)
    3. Metoclopramide (Reglan)
    4. Dicyclomine (Bentyl)

20. Which agents are used in the treatment of GERD and PUD to reduce the secretion of saliva, hydrochloric acid, pepsin, and bile? *(503-504)*
    1. Antispasmodics
    2. Proton pump inhibitors
    3. Antacids
    4. Histamine receptor antagonists

Identify interventions that incorporate pharmacologic and nonpharmacologic treatments for an individual with stomach disorders.

21. Which statement does the nurse include when teaching a patient about antacid therapy for the treatment of peptic ulcer disease? *(496)*
    1. "Antacids take at least 6 weeks to become effective."
    2. "Antacid tablets do not contain enough antacid to be effective in treating this disease."
    3. "Excessive use of magnesium antacids results in constipation."
    4. "A common complaint of patients using large quantities of calcium carbonate antacids is diarrhea."
22. A patient with a history of chronic renal failure is on high-dose cimetidine (Tagamet) therapy for the treatment of a duodenal ulcer. It is most important for the nurse to assess the patient for which adverse effect of this therapy? *(498)*
    1. Dizziness
    2. Constipation
    3. Disorientation
    4. Diarrhea
23. When teaching the patient in the scenario about the use of antacids as part of the treatment for GERD, which statements does the nurse include? *(Select all that apply.)* *(496)*
    1. "Maalox is an example of a low-sodium antacid."
    2. "Use of an antacid with large amounts of magnesium usually results in constipation."
    3. "Calcium carbonate and sodium bicarbonate may cause rebound hyperacidity."
    4. "Patients with renal failure should not use large quantities of antacids containing magnesium."
    5. "Antacid tablets should be used only for patients with occasional indigestion or heartburn."

Drugs Used to Treat Nausea and Vomiting

Answer Key: Textbook page references are provided as a guide for answering these questions. A complete answer key is provided to your instructor.

MATCHING
Match the drug on the right with the drug class on the left.

	Drug Class		Drug Name
1. _____	dopamine antagonists	a.	dimenhydrinate
2. _____	serotonin antagonists	b.	aprepitant
3. _____	anticholinergic agents	c.	prochlorperazine
4. _____	corticosteroids	d.	lorazepam
5. _____	benzodiazepines	e.	dronabinol
6. _____	cannabinoids	f.	dexamethasone
7. _____	neurokinin-1 receptor antagonists	g.	ondansetron

REVIEW QUESTIONS

Scenario: A 26-year-old pregnant woman came in to the outpatient clinic complaining about severe persistent vomiting for the past several weeks. She states that it is impossible to keep anything down and now she is getting weak.

Describe the six common causes of nausea and vomiting.

8. Nausea and vomiting symptoms associated with motion sickness are thought to result from stimulation of the: *(508)*
   1. diaphragm.
   2. sensory receptors on the tongue and soft palate.
   3. cerebral cortex.
   4. labyrinth system of the ear.
9. The nurse knows that some of the most common causes of nausea and vomiting include: *(Select all that apply.) (508)*
   1. thyroid disorders.
   2. pain.
   3. drug therapy.
   4. gastrointestinal disorders.
   5. pregnancy.
10. The patient in the scenario has which condition in which starvation, dehydration, and acidosis are superimposed on the vomiting, requiring hospitalization? *(509)*
    1. Drug toxicity
    2. Regurgitation
    3. Hyperemesis gravidarum
    4. Delayed emesis
11. Patients who have cancer and are undergoing treatment with gamma rays and chemotherapy may develop the adverse effect of nausea and vomiting called: *(Select all that apply.) (509)*
    1. delayed emesis.
    2. psychogenic vomiting.
    3. chemotherapy-induced nausea and vomiting.
    4. postoperative nausea and vomiting.
    5. radiation-induced nausea and vomiting.

Discuss the three types of nausea associated with chemotherapy and the nursing considerations.

12. Chemotherapy and radiation therapy used for cancer treatment are associated with different types of adverse effects. Nausea and vomiting top the list as the most unpleasant, which can trigger a conditioned response known as: *(509)*
    1. delayed emesis.
    2. anticipatory nausea and vomiting.
    3. hyperemesis gravidarum.
    4. regurgitation.

13. The various ways that patients are treated with antiemetics to prevent chemotherapy-induced nausea and vomiting are to: *(Select all that apply.)* **(511)**
    1. use a combination of antiemetic agents.
    2. use the least emetogenic agent for chemotherapy.
    3. administer antiemetics prior to chemotherapy.
    4. encourage the use of over-the-counter herbal supplements for treatment.
    5. continue the antiemetic therapy for several weeks following chemotherapy.
14. Which antineoplastic agents are considered a high emetic risk? *(Select all that apply.)* **(509)**
    1. Carmustine
    2. Carboplatin
    3. Cetuximab
    4. Cisplatin
    5. Cyclophosphamide
15. The nurse explained to the patient who recently underwent radiation therapy the factors that influence radiation-induced nausea and vomiting, which include the: *(Select all that apply.)* **(510)**
    1. treatment site.
    2. field exposure.
    3. dose of radiation delivered.
    4. number of cancer cells radiated.
    5. previous development of nausea and vomiting.

Identify the therapeutic classes of antiemetics.

16. The nurse was talking with a patient who mentioned he heard that marijuana is used for nausea now and would like some for his symptoms. The best response by the nurse would be: **(522)**
    1. "You cannot have any marijuana. It is illegal."
    2. "The active ingredient in marijuana has been made into a medication that your doctor may prescribe for you."
    3. "I will have to ask your doctor if it would be okay for you to have any."
    4. "I heard it does not really help patients who are nauseated. I would not recommend it."
17. Most antiemetic agents used to reduce nausea and vomiting from motion sickness are chemically related to: **(510)**

1. analgesics.
2. ginger.
3. antihistamines.
4. *Ginkgo biloba.*

18. Which antiemetic medications would be of benefit to give to the patient in the scenario? *(Select all that apply.)* **(511)**
    1. Benzodiazepines (e.g., lorazepam, diazepam)
    2. Corticosteroids (e.g., dexamethasone)
    3. Antihistamines (e.g., diphenhydramine, meclizine)
    4. Phenothiazines (e.g., promethazine, prochlorperazine)
    5. Serotonin antagonists (e.g., granisetron, ondansetron)

Discuss the scheduling of antiemetics for maximum benefit.

19. The nurse was discussing the best timing for cyclizine (Marezine) with a patient taking it for motion sickness, and knows the patient needs more teaching after hearing which response? **(518, 521)**
    1. "I will take this drug 30 to 45 minutes before I need to drive any long distance."
    2. "I will take this drug when I start to feel nauseated."
    3. "For the best effect from this drug, I need to take it prior to travel by plane."
    4. "This drug has fewer side effects than Benadryl."
20. For patients undergoing chemotherapy, the nurse knows that if the acute emesis and nausea are controlled completely, the possibility of what is decreased significantly? **(511)**
    1. Motion sickness
    2. Psychogenic vomiting
    3. Hyperemesis gravidarum
    4. Delayed emesis
21. When should antiemetic agents be administered to be considered most effective? **(510)**
    1. Before the onset of nausea
    2. After nausea has occurred
    3. After vomiting has occurred
    4. It does not matter

	chapter
# Drugs Used to Treat Constipation and Diarrhea	# 34

Answer Key: Textbook page references are provided as a guide for answering these questions. A complete answer key is provided to your instructor.

MATCHING

Match the drug class on the right to the drug name on the left. Drug classes can be used more than once.

Drug Name

1. _____ lactulose
2. _____ docusate sodium
3. _____ bismuth subsalicylate
4. _____ atropine
5. _____ bisacodyl
6. _____ loperamide
7. _____ polyethylene glycol

Drug Class

a. laxatives
b. antidiarrheal agents

REVIEW QUESTIONS

Scenario: A 72-year-old male patient admitted to the hospital with recent mental status changes, gastroesophageal reflux disease (GERD), and symptoms of gastric outlet obstruction was being managed with a nasogastric (NG) tube. He also had a history of Crohn's disease with a bowel resection resulting in an ileostomy and was experiencing high output from the ileostomy.

Explain the meaning of "normal" bowel habits and describe the underlying causes of constipation.

8. The nurse was explaining to a patient what was meant by "normal" bowel habits, stating: *(526)*
   1. "Sometimes it is normal to have 2 or 3 bowel movements per week."
   2. "Daily bowel movements are necessary for good health."
   3. "You need to start worrying about unhealthy bowel movements when the stool becomes soft and brown."
   4. "Using laxatives or enemas daily should be just fine."
9. A patient asked the nurse for some advice on how to prevent constipation that was bothering him lately. Important responses include: *(Select all that apply.)* *(526)*

   1. "What type of diet do you follow? One with plenty of fruits and vegetables and limited cheese and yogurt should help."
   2. "Tell me about your daily activity level. Being physically active helps eliminate problems."
   3. "Can you tell me about how much water you drink every day? It is important to keep well-hydrated."
   4. "Do you have any history of diseases of the stomach?"
   5. "Tell me about the medications you are taking. Certain types of drugs can cause constipation."
10. Which of these conditions may contribute to constipation for patients? *(Select all that apply.)* *(526)*
    1. Hyperthyroidism
    2. Anemia
    3. Hypothyroidism
    4. Tumors of the bowel
    5. Crohn's disease

Identify the mechanism of action for the different classes of laxatives, and describe medical conditions in which laxatives should not be used.

11. What is the mechanism of action of stimulant laxatives? *(529)*
    1. They draw water into the intestine from surrounding tissues by means of hypertonic compounds.

2. They act directly on the intestine, causing irritation that promotes peristalsis and evacuation.
3. They add lubrication to the intestinal wall and soften the stool.
4. They draw water into the stool, causing it to soften.

12. Which statement does the nurse include when teaching a patient about the use of osmotic laxatives? *(529)*
    1. "These agents usually work within 8 to 12 hours."
    2. "These agents should be used only intermittently because chronic use may cause loss of normal bowel function."
    3. "Osmotic laxatives work by making the stool softer."
    4. "Osmotic laxatives restore normal intestinal flora."

13. What is the mechanism of action of lubricant laxatives? *(530)*
    1. They lubricate the intestinal wall and soften the stool to allow a smooth passage of fecal contents.
    2. They increase peristalsis.
    3. They draw more water into the stool.
    4. They increase bulk in the stool to stimulate peristalsis.

14. Which statements about bulk-forming laxatives are true? *(Select all that apply.)* *(530)*
    1. They are generally considered to be the drug of choice for people who are incapacitated and need a laxative regularly.
    2. They may be used in the treatment of patients with irritable bowel syndrome.
    3. They are used to treat certain types of diarrhea.
    4. Adequate volumes of water must be taken with bulk-forming laxatives.
    5. They are used to relieve acute constipation.

15. What is the mechanism of action of fecal softeners? *(527)*
    1. They draw water into the stool, causing it to soften.
    2. They add bulk to the stool.
    3. They stimulate peristalsis.
    4. They lubricate the intestines.

16. In which situations should laxatives not be used? *(Select all that apply.)* *(527)*
    1. Patients with nausea, vomiting, or fever
    2. Patients with severe pain or discomfort
    3. Patients taking medicines that cause diarrhea
    4. Patients with constipation
    5. Patients with success in the past using laxatives

Cite nine causes of diarrhea.

17. Which conditions predispose the patient to developing diarrhea? *(Select all that apply.)* *(527)*
    1. Hypothyroidism
    2. Anemia
    3. Hyperthyroidism

4. Crohn's disease
5. Enzyme deficiencies

18. Diet is an important consideration for patients who have developed diarrhea. The nurse educates the patient on which food items to avoid to prevent diarrhea? *(Select all that apply.)* *(527)*
    1. Spicy foods
    2. Deep-fat fried foods
    3. Drinking tap water when on vacation in another country
    4. Fresh oysters
    5. Cheese and yogurt

19. Which condition did the patient in the scenario have that is an example of a common cause of diarrhea? *(527)*
    1. Mental status changes
    2. GERD
    3. Gastric outlet obstruction
    4. GI surgery

Differentiate between locally acting and systemically acting antidiarrheal agents.

20. Systemically acting antidiarrheal agents such as loperamide (Imodium) work by: *(533)*
    1. absorbing nutrients, water, and electrolytes and leaving a formed stool.
    2. increasing peristalsis and GI motility via the autonomic nervous system.
    3. decreasing peristalsis and GI motility via the autonomic nervous system.
    4. promoting the expulsion of formed stool.

21. Locally acting antidiarrheal agents such as bismuth subsalicylate (Pepto-Bismol) work by: *(Select all that apply.)* *(533)*
    1. adsorbing irritants or bacteria from the GI tract that cause diarrhea.
    2. absorbing excess water to produce a formed stool.
    3. decreasing peristalsis and GI motility.
    4. reducing pain and irritation associated with diarrhea.
    5. increasing peristalsis and GI motility.

22. Which antidiarrheal agent has the potential to cause a hypertensive crisis when administered with a monoamine oxidase inhibitor? *(533)*
    1. Bismuth subsalicylate (Pepto-Bismol)
    2. *Lactobacillus acidophilus* (Lactinex)
    3. Loperamide (Imodium)
    4. Diphenoxylate with atropine (Lomotil)

Describe nursing assessments needed to evaluate the patient's state of hydration when suffering from either constipation or dehydration, and identify electrolytes that should be monitored whenever prolonged or severe diarrhea is present.

23. The patient in the scenario was at risk for which condition? *(527)*
    1. Hyperkalemia
    2. Dehydration

3. Fluid volume excess
4. Hypernatremia

24. The nurse will need to monitor which laboratory values for the patient in the scenario? *(Select all that apply.)* *(528)*
    1. Potassium
    2. Creatinine
    3. Bicarbonate
    4. Alkaline phosphate
    5. Chloride

25. Assessments of the patient made by the nurse to determine hydration status include checking: *(Select all that apply.)* *(528)*
    1. skin turgor.
    2. mucous membranes.
    3. weight.
    4. urine output.
    5. appetite.

Cite conditions that generally respond favorably to antidiarrheal agents.

26. Which patient conditions generally respond positively to antidiarrheal agents? *(Select all that apply.)* *(532)*

1. Severe constipation
2. Following GI surgery
3. Traveler's diarrhea
4. Small bowel obstruction
5. Inflammatory bowel disease

27. A patient experiencing diarrhea with extreme pain would likely receive which drug to inhibit peristalsis and assist with the pain? *(533)*
    1. Diphenoxylate with atropine (Lomotil)
    2. Opium (Paregoric)
    3. Loperamide (Imodium)
    4. Difenoxin with atropine (Motofen)

28. Which patient is most likely to benefit from the effects of a laxative? *(528)*
    1. 27-year-old who has colitis
    2. 49-year-old diagnosed with appendicitis
    3. 34-year-old paraplegic
    4. 65-year-old with gastritis

Drugs Used to Treat Diabetes Mellitus

chapter
35

Answer Key: Textbook page references are provided as a guide for answering these questions. A complete answer key is provided to your instructor.

MATCHING
Match the drug class on the right with the drug name on the left.

Drug Name

1. _____ metformin (Glucophage)
2. _____ exenatide (Byetta)
3. _____ canagliflozin (Invokana)
4. _____ repaglinide (Prandin)
5. _____ aspart (NovoLog)
6. _____ rosiglitazone (Avandia)
7. _____ glimepiride (Amaryl)
8. _____ sitagliptin (Januvia)
9. _____ acarbose (Precose)

Drug Class

a. insulin
b. sulfonylureas
c. meglitinides
d. biguanide
e. thiazolidinediones
f. alpha-glucosidase inhibitors
g. glucagon-like peptide-1 agonists
h. dipeptidyl peptidase-4 inhibitors
i. sodium-glucose cotransporter 2 inhibitors

REVIEW QUESTIONS

Scenario: A 73-year-old female patient came to the outpatient clinic complaining that her left great toe was painful, swollen, and red. She has a history of type 2 diabetes mellitus, asthma, atrial fibrillation, peripheral arterial disease, gastric bypass surgery, and neuropathy.

Identify normal fasting blood glucose levels and differentiate between the symptoms of type 1 and type 2 diabetes mellitus.

10. Type 1 diabetes mellitus, caused by an autoimmune destruction of the beta cells in the pancreas, also has characteristics that differentiate it from type 2, such as: *(Select all that apply.)* **(536)**
    1. it is thought to be immune-mediated.
    2. it requires the administration of insulin.
    3. it is associated with increased frequency of infections and loss of weight and strength.
    4. its symptoms are characterized by polydipsia, polyphagia, and polyuria.
    5. it can be controlled by eliminating sugar from the diet.
11. Diabetes mellitus is a group of diseases characterized by what pathology? *(Select all that apply.)* **(535)**

1. Any plasma glucose level >126 mg/dL
2. Decrease in appetite and urination
3. Fasting plasma glucose >126 mg/dL
4. Impairment of insulin secretion
5. Abnormalities in fat, carbohydrate, and protein metabolism

12. Type 2 diabetes mellitus is characterized by which conditions? *(Select all that apply.)* **(536)**
    1. Type 2 causes an increase in glucose produced by the liver.
    2. Type 2 is caused by a decrease in beta cell activity.
    3. Type 2 causes an increase in glycogen stored by the liver.
    4. Type 2 has fasting glucose levels <126 mg/dL.
    5. Type 2 is caused by insulin resistance syndrome.

13. Which statements does the nurse include when teaching health promotion activities to a patient with type 2 diabetes mellitus? *(Select all that apply.)* **(546)**
    1. "If you feel sick, cut your insulin dose by half."
    2. "If your blood glucose is greater than 240 mg/dL, you should test your urine for ketones."

3. "Notify your primary healthcare provider immediately if you are unable to keep anything down."
4. "Extra insulin is often needed to meet the demands of illness, so be aware of the development of hyperglycemia, which is common in patients with acute illness, injury, or surgery."
5. "Store unused insulin in the freezer."

Identify the major nursing considerations associated with the management of the patient with diabetes (e.g., nutritional evaluation, dietary prescription, activity and exercise, and psychological considerations).

14. The medical nutrition therapy recommended by the ADA to help maintain dietary restrictions for patients trying to control their diabetes by diet include: *(Select all that apply.)* *(543-544)*
    1. measuring food for balanced portions.
    2. not omitting meals or between-meal snacks.
    3. eliminating all sugar from the diet.
    4. increasing exercise when eating more.
    5. keeping in mind food preferences and economic status.

15. The nurse was discussing how to count carbohydrates to determine the amount of insulin to be administered with each meal. Which statement made by the patient indicates a need for further teaching? *(544)*
    1. "I can have between 1500 and 2000 calories every day."
    2. "I should get approximately 45% to 65% of my calories from carbohydrates."
    3. "I should get approximately 20% to 35% of my calories from fat."
    4. "I should get approximately 25% to 45% of my calories from protein sources."

16. The aims of dietary control for type 2 diabetics include: *(Select all that apply.)* *(538)*
    1. prevention of excessive postprandial hyperglycemia.
    2. maintenance of ideal body weight.
    3. prevention of hypoglycemia.
    4. elimination of cholesterol from the diet.
    5. reducing elevated cholesterol and triglyceride levels.

17. The nurse is educating the patient in the scenario about activity and exercise and because of her neuropathy, recommended which types of exercises? *(Select all that apply.)* *(545)*
    1. Walking
    2. Bicycling
    3. Swimming
    4. Rowing
    5. Treadmill

Compare the signs, symptoms, and management of hypoglycemia and hyperglycemia.

18. A nurse was discussing the symptoms and management of hypoglycemia with the patient in the scenario. Which statement by the patient would indicate further education is needed? *(546)*
    1. "When I start to feel hungry, get a headache, and my vision blurs, I know I am getting hypoglycemic."
    2. "When I start to feel hypoglycemic, I should drink some fruit juice with sugar added."
    3. "I can control the episodes of hypoglycemia by eating at regular times and watching what I eat."
    4. "I know I am getting hypoglycemic when I start to feel thirsty several hours after eating a large meal."

19. A nurse caring for a diabetic patient noted the following symptoms: increased thirst, headache, nausea and vomiting, rapid pulse, and shallow respirations. This could represent what condition? *(546)*
    1. Insulin overdose
    2. Hypoglycemia
    3. Hyperglycemia
    4. Paresthesias

20. Which drug classification when taken with insulin is most likely to induce hypoglycemia, and/or mask many of the symptoms of hypoglycemia? *(554)*
    1. Corticosteroids
    2. Calcium channel blockers
    3. Benzodiazepines
    4. Beta-adrenergic blocking agents

21. Which are considered causes of hyperglycemia? *(Select all that apply.)* *(546)*
    1. Overeating
    2. Vomiting
    3. Acute illness
    4. Infections
    5. Diarrhea

Describe the action and use of insulin to control diabetes mellitus.

22. Which type of insulin has an onset of 1 to 2 hours, peaks within 4 to 12 hours, and lasts from 16 to 28 hours? *(551)*
    1. Intermediate-acting
    2. Short-acting
    3. Rapid-acting
    4. Long-acting

23. When is the ideal time to administer rapid-acting insulin? *(549)*
    1. 30 minutes before a meal
    2. 30 minutes after a meal
    3. 10 to 15 minutes before a meal
    4. 10 to 15 minutes after a meal

24. What are the major advantages of insulin glargine and detemir? *(552)*

1. They are given in the morning for the best effect.
2. They do not result in large fluctuations in insulin levels.
3. They will decrease the blood sugar level rapidly.
4. They peak within 30 minutes.

25. The nurse is educating the patient in the scenario on the use of the rapid-acting insulin aspart while she is in the hospital and knows more education is needed after the patient makes which remark? *(552)*
    1. "So as I understand it, I will only be on insulin while I am in the hospital to control my blood sugars."
    2. "The insulin aspart that I am receiving is a rapid-acting one that peaks in 1-3 hours."
    3. "I need to have my blood sugar checked four times a day with this insulin."
    4. "This insulin has an onset of 1-2 hours and lasts 16 hours."

Discuss the action and use of oral hypoglycemic agents to control diabetes mellitus.

26. Which class of oral hypoglycemic agent lowers blood sugar in diabetic patients by increasing the sensitivity of muscle and fat tissue to insulin? *(559)*
    1. Meglitinides
    2. Thiazolidinediones
    3. Sulfonylureas
    4. Amylinomimetics

27. Which patient is most likely to benefit from treatment with sulfonylurea oral hypoglycemic agents? *(555)*
    1. Diabetic type 1
    2. Diabetic type 2, not controlled by diet and exercise
    3. Newly diagnosed diabetic 18-month-old infant
    4. Diabetic on 60 units of NPH insulin a day

28. Alpha-glucosidase inhibitors are an example of the type of oral hypoglycemic agent that works by lowering blood sugar in diabetic patients by: *(560)*
    1. inhibiting digestive enzymes that result in delayed glucose absorption.
    2. increasing the sensitivity of muscle and fat tissue to insulin.
    3. enhancing insulin secretion and suppressing glucagon secretion from the liver.
    4. stimulating the release of insulin from the beta cells of the pancreas.

29. The nurse realized the patient in the scenario was having difficulty with her diabetic management because her A1C level result was: *(541)*
    1. 5.3.
    2. 6.0.
    3. 8.5.
    4. 4.0.

30. The patient in the scenario was being started on acarbose (Precose) and glipizide (Glucotrol). Which statement by the nurse would be included in the discussion of adverse effects from these drugs? *(556)*
    1. "You may experience nausea, vomiting, and abdominal cramps, in which case you must stop taking these drugs immediately."
    2. "If you develop a rash with itching, don't worry; it should get better eventually."
    3. "You may develop abdominal cramps and diarrhea, but these symptoms will resolve with continued use of your medications."
    4. "You will need to change your diet with these drugs and consume greater portions of protein."

31. It is important for the nurse to inform female patients with diabetes that an alternative method of birth control should be used when taking which oral hypoglycemic agent? *(560)*
    1. Miglitol (Glyset)
    2. Glyburide (Glynase)
    3. Pramlintide (Symlin)
    4. Pioglitazone (Actos)

Discuss the educational needs for patients with complications from diabetes (e.g., symptoms of microvascular and macrovascular complications).

32. What signs and symptoms of microvascular complications of peripheral vascular disease may diabetic patients develop? *(Select all that apply.)* *(547)*
    1. Ulcers may develop on legs and feet.
    2. Circulation may become impaired with decreased peripheral pulses.
    3. Reddish-blue discoloration may appear over legs and feet.
    4. Temperature of the skin in the feet and legs may be cool to the touch.
    5. Urinary tract infections increase in frequency.

33. The patient in the scenario had examples of complications from her diabetes. Identify those conditions. *(Select all that apply.)* *(538)*
    1. Peripheral arterial disease
    2. Asthma
    3. Neuropathy
    4. Cellulitis of the great toe
    5. Atrial fibrillation

34. The major macrovascular complications of diabetes are associated with atherosclerotic disease of the middle to large arteries often leading to myocardial infarction and stroke, as well as: *(Select all that apply.)* *(538)*
    1. renal disease leading to end-stage renal disease and dialysis.
    2. amputations of the lower extremities.
    3. ototoxicity leading to hearing loss.
    4. retinopathy leading to blindness.
    5. peripheral arterial disease leading to nonhealing ulcers and infections.

35. The new diabetic patient needs instructions on how to manage diabetes, as well as any special equipment that is utilized, such as: *(Select all that apply.)* *(548)*
    1. an insulin pump.
    2. a self-monitoring glucose machine.
    3. syringes.
    4. a walker.
    5. a computer.

Drugs Used to Treat Thyroid Disease

Answer Key: Textbook page references are provided as a guide for answering these questions. A complete answer key is provided to your instructor.

MATCHING

Match the definition on the right with the key term on the left. Definitions may be used more than once.

	Key Term		Definition
1. _____	myxedema	a.	congenital hypothyroidism
2. _____	cretinism	b.	excess production of thyroid hormones
		c.	thyroid hormone
3. _____	hyperthyroidism	d.	inadequate thyroid hormone production
4. _____	thyrotoxicosis	e.	hypothyroidism during adult life
5. _____	hypothyroidism	f.	excessive formation of thyroid hormones and their secretion into the circulatory system
6. _____	triiodothyronine		
7. _____	thyroxine		

REVIEW QUESTIONS

Scenario: A 48-year-old female patient came to an outpatient clinic complaining of increased fatigue and unexplained weight gain. She mentioned that she was beginning to have problems with constipation and felt cold all the time.

Describe the function of the thyroid gland.

8. What body functions are regulated by the thyroid gland? *(Select all that apply.)* **(571)**
   1. Pulmonary function
   2. Cardiovascular function
   3. Carbohydrate, protein, and lipid metabolism
   4. Growth and reproduction
   5. Thermal regulation
9. The large, reddish, ductless gland located on either side of the trachea produces which hormones? *(Select all that apply.)* **(571)**
   1. Triiodothyronine
   2. Thyrotropin
   3. Thyroxine
   4. Thyroid-stimulating hormone
   5. Thyroglobulin
10. The hypothalamus and the anterior pituitary gland regulate the thyroid gland by secreting which hormones? *(Select all that apply.)* **(571)**
    1. Thyrotropin-releasing hormone
    2. Thyroid-stimulating hormone
    3. Thyroid-releasing hormone
    4. Thyroxine
    5. Triiodothyronine

Identify the two classes of drugs used to treat thyroid disease.

11. When drug therapy is prescribed for patients with hyperthyroidism, they may be given: **(572)**
    1. levothyroxine.
    2. methimazole.
    3. liotrix.
    4. liothyronine.
12. The antithyroid drugs work by interfering with the: *(Select all that apply.)* **(572)**
    1. release of thyroid hormones from the thyroid gland.
    2. formation of the hormones produced by the thyroid gland.
    3. metabolic requirements of the body.
    4. follicles surrounding the thyroid gland.
    5. release of TSH from the pituitary gland.
13. The patient in the scenario needs to be started on a thyroid replacement hormone such as: **(575)**
    1. methimazole.
    2. propylthiouracil.
    3. levothyroxine.
    4. thyroglobulin.

Describe the signs, symptoms, treatment, and nursing interventions associated with hypothyroidism and identify the drug of choice for hypothyroidism.

14. What focused assessments should be performed by the nurse for the patient in the scenario? *(Select all that apply.)* *(573)*
    1. Cardiovascular—pulse and blood pressure
    2. Neurologic—nervousness and agitation
    3. Gastrointestinal—constipation
    4. Sensory—presence of exophthalmos
    5. Respiratory—rate and effort of breathing

15. A patient with hypothyroidism may require what dietary changes? *(573)*
    1. Increase in fats
    2. Decrease in calories
    3. Increase in calories
    4. Decrease in fats

16. The patient in the scenario was diagnosed with hypothyroidism and the nurse gave which instructions to her regarding this diagnosis and treatment? *(Select all that apply.)* *(574)*
    1. "You should take your Synthroid with food around lunchtime."
    2. "You will need to start taking thyroid hormones for the treatment of this condition."
    3. "You may find that you will be more comfortable in a warm environment."
    4. "You need to be aware of the signs of hyperthyroidism, which can be caused by too much thyroid medication."
    5. "The dosages of this thyroid medication start high and then gradually decrease in amount until you reach your daily maintenance dose."

Describe the signs, symptoms, treatments, and nursing interventions associated with hyperthyroidism.

17. Which disorders may cause hyperactivity of the thyroid gland that results in hyperthyroidism? *(Select all that apply.)* *(572)*
    1. Thyroid carcinoma
    2. Graves' disease
    3. Tumors of the pituitary gland
    4. Nodular goiter
    5. Myxedema

18. Which manifestation does the nurse expect to find upon assessing a patient who has been diagnosed with hyperthyroidism? *(Select all that apply.)* *(572)*
    1. Rapid, bounding pulse
    2. Nervousness and agitation
    3. Weight loss
    4. Puffy face
    5. Insomnia

19. The primary therapeutic outcome for hyperthyroidism is a gradual return to normal thyroid metabolic function expected from which drugs? *(Select all that apply.)* *(577)*
    1. Levothyroxine
    2. Liothyronine
    3. Propylthiouracil
    4. Liotrix
    5. Methimazole

20. The nurse has been teaching a patient diagnosed with hyperthyroidism about proper nutritional habits to follow. Which patient statement indicates a need for further teaching? *(573)*
    1. "I will limit my fluid intake to three 8-ounce glasses of water a day."
    2. "I will eat a high-calorie diet, about 4000 to 5000 calories a day."
    3. "I will drink decaffeinated cola."
    4. "I will avoid chocolate."

21. The patient in the scenario was on digoxin (Lanoxin) and needed to be started on levothyroxine (Synthroid) for the treatment of her hypothyroidism. The nurse explains which interaction between these drugs? *(576)*
    1. "You will most likely have to adjust your dosages of Synthroid every week."
    2. "You will most likely require an increased dose of digoxin."
    3. "You will most likely require a decreased dose of digoxin."
    4. "You will most likely require increasing dosages of Synthroid."

22. The nurse is instructing a patient recently diagnosed with hyperthyroidism on what activity is allowed. Which statement by the patient would indicate that further teaching is needed? *(574)*
    1. "I will need to pace myself with activities so that I do not get too tired."
    2. "I know that I should increase my activities every week even if I have pain."
    3. "If I feel weak and tired, I should not try to overdo it as far as exercising."
    4. "I understand that I should continue to be active but careful with overdoing exercise."

Discuss the drug interactions associated with thyroid hormones and antithyroid medicines.

23. Radioactive iodine is used in the treatment of hyperthyroidism because this drug will: *(576)*
    1. cause the thyroid gland to radiate a soft, warm glow.
    2. absorb all of the excess thyroid hormone that is circulating in the blood.
    3. be absorbed into the thyroid gland and destroy the hyperactive tissue.
    4. increase the circulating thyrotropin-releasing hormone.

24. When administering iodine-131 (^{131}I) to a patient, what actions does the nurse take? *(Select all that apply.)* *(577)*
    1. Adds the medication to water and has the patient swallow it

2. Wears latex gloves when administering the drug
3. Avoids spilling the medication
4. Changes the patient's bedding after each dose
5. Maintains hazardous medication precautions when working with the drug

25. Patients who require more than one dose of iodine-131 generally have to wait an interval of at least: *(576)*
    1. 1 month between doses.
    2. 2 months between doses.
    3. 3 months between doses.
    4. 4 months between doses.

26. Dietary requirements for patients who have hyperthyroidism include: *(574)*
    1. fluid restriction.
    2. decreased caloric intake.
    3. increased bran products, fruits, and fresh vegetables.
    4. increased caloric intake.

27. A patient with dramatic weight loss and rapid, bounding pulse may be suffering from: *(572)*
    1. myxedema.
    2. hypothyroidism.
    3. hyperthyroidism.
    4. cretinism.

Cite the actions of propylthiouracil on the synthesis of T_3 and T_4.

28. Which are the types of conditions that respond favorably to the use of iodine-131? *(Select all that apply.)* *(576)*
    1. Patients who need long-term treatment of hyperthyroidism
    2. Patients who need short-term treatment before subtotal thyroidectomy
    3. Older patients who are beyond the childbearing years
    4. Patients with recurrent hyperthyroidism after previous thyroid surgery
    5. Patients with unusually small thyroid glands

29. Propylthiouracil (PTU, Propacil) and methimazole (Tapazole) are used to treat hyperthyroidism, and work in which way? *(577)*
    1. They absorb the circulating T_3 and T_4.
    2. They block the synthesis of T_3 and T_4.
    3. They destroy any T_3 and T_4 already produced.
    4. They inactivate the circulating T_3 and T_4.

30. The nurse will need to monitor which laboratory studies for patients who are taking the antithyroid medications propylthiouracil (PTU, Propacil) and methimazole (Tapazole)? *(Select all that apply.)* *(577)*
    1. Complete blood count with differential
    2. TSH
    3. Protime
    4. Thyroid hormone
    5. BUN

Corticosteroids

chapter

37

Answer Key: Textbook page references are provided as a guide for answering these questions. A complete answer key is provided to your instructor.

MATCHING

Match the brand name drug on the right with the generic drug name on the left.

	Generic Drug Name		Brand Name Drug
1.	_____ dexamethasone	a.	Kenalog
2.	_____ budesonide	b.	Maxidex
		c.	Cortef
3.	_____ mometasone	d.	Prelone
4.	_____ hydrocortisone	e.	Solu-Medrol
5.	_____ methylprednisolone	f.	Nasonex
6.	_____ prednisolone	g.	Pulmicort
7.	_____ triamcinolone		

REVIEW QUESTIONS

Scenario: A 75-year-old male patient was admitted to the hospital for respiratory failure and was diagnosed with pneumonia. He had a history of chronic obstructive pulmonary disease (COPD), osteoporosis, hypothyroidism, depression, congestive heart failure (CHF), coronary artery disease with previous bypass grafts, and rheumatoid arthritis. His medication list included levothyroxine, metoprolol, prednisone, duloxetine, acetaminophen, senna, and oxycodone.

Discuss the normal actions of mineralocorticoids and glucocorticoids in the body.

8. The adrenal gland secretes hormones that maintain fluid and electrolyte balance and regulate metabolism of carbohydrates, fats, and protein. These hormones are known collectively as: *(580)*
   1. mineralocorticoids.
   2. glucocorticoids.
   3. corticosteroids.
   4. aldosterone.
9. The corticosteroids are used to regulate the body's metabolism. Which laboratory tests are to be monitored for patients receiving these medications? *(Select all that apply.) (581)*
   1. Hemoglobin
   2. Protime
   3. Glucose
   4. Potassium
   5. Sodium
10. The nurse has been teaching a patient with an exacerbation of rheumatoid arthritis about the use of glucocorticoids. Which statement by the patient indicates a need for further instruction? *(584)*
    1. "This drug has cured my disease."
    2. "This drug is relieving the inflammation associated with rheumatoid arthritis."
    3. "My fingers will not change back to normal shape due to this drug treatment."
    4. "I must be aware that I am more susceptible to infections when taking these drugs."

Cite the disease states caused by hyposecretion of the adrenal gland.

11. Which drug is given to patients who have a hyposecretion of the adrenal gland known as Addison's disease? *(583)*
    1. Fludrocortisone
    2. Dexamethasone
    3. Methylprednisolone
    4. Betamethasone
12. When patients are on the drug triamcinolone (a glucocorticoid), the medication may be in the form of: *(Select all that apply.) (585)*
    1. topical creams and ointments.

2. tablets and oral syrups.
3. shampoos, gels, and oils.
4. lotions and sprays.
5. aerosols and inhalants.

13. Glucocorticoids must be used with caution in patients with which disorders? *(Select all that apply.)* *(586)*
    1. Type 1 diabetes mellitus
    2. Type 2 diabetes mellitus
    3. Upper respiratory infections
    4. Severe hay fever
    5. Mental disturbances

Identify the baseline assessments needed for a patient receiving corticosteroids.

14. What baseline assessments by the nurse should be completed for patients taking any type of corticosteroids? *(Select all that apply.)* *(580)*
    1. Daily weights
    2. Pulse checks in supine and sitting position
    3. Intake and output
    4. Sodium, potassium, and blood glucose
    5. Signs and symptoms of infection

15. What is the priority assessment for the nurse to make when caring for a patient on fludrocortisone (Florinef) therapy for Addison's disease? *(584)*
    1. Allergic reactions
    2. Hyponatremia
    3. Hypokalemia
    4. Hypotension

16. The nurse is assessing a patient taking glucocorticoids for the treatment of rheumatoid arthritis. Which findings are indications that the medication is exerting its desired effect? *(Select all that apply.)* *(584)*
    1. Pain relief
    2. Elevated sedimentation rates
    3. Normalization of preexisting joint deformities
    4. Increased energy
    5. Relief of swelling

17. Which signs of dehydration need to be assessed by the nurse when patients are receiving corticosteroids? *(Select all that apply.)* *(581)*
    1. Delayed capillary refill
    2. Dry mucous membranes
    3. Peripheral edema
    4. Bounding pulses
    5. Poor skin turgor

Discuss the clinical uses and potential adverse effects associated with corticosteroids.

18. A nurse was teaching a patient with Addison's disease about the condition and how it is treated. Which statement by the patient indicates that further teaching is needed? *(582)*

1. "I understand that my adrenal glands are not producing enough of the hormone needed to regulate water and electrolytes."
2. "I understand that I need to watch my weight and report significant changes."
3. "I know that when I go get my blood drawn, the most important test reported is the level of calcium."
4. "I know I cannot stop taking these hormones unless I am under a healthcare provider's care."

19. Which types of illnesses or conditions are frequently treated with glucocorticoids? *(Select all that apply.)* *(584)*
    1. Nausea and vomiting associated with chemotherapy
    2. Inflammatory conditions
    3. Allergies
    4. Autoimmune disorders that require an immunosuppressant
    5. Bacterial infections

20. What adverse effects does the nurse need to be aware of in patients who are receiving glucocorticoids? *(Select all that apply.)* *(581)*
    1. Hyperglycemia
    2. Electrolyte imbalances and fluid accumulation
    3. Hypoglycemia
    4. Increased susceptibility to infection
    5. Peptic ulcer formation

21. The nurse was teaching a patient about precautions necessary when receiving steroid therapy. Further education is needed when the patient makes which statement? *(582-583)*
    1. "I understand that if I start to develop edema in my feet, ankles, or legs I need to notify my healthcare provider."
    2. "I will need to get an identification bracelet to wear at all times."
    3. "I know I should not suddenly stop taking these medications."
    4. "I can expect that a weight gain of 2 pounds in 2 days is normal."

22. The drug prednisone (a glucocorticoid) has an anti-inflammatory effect and is used for the patient in the scenario for which diagnosis? *(584)*
    1. Hypothyroidism
    2. Rheumatoid arthritis
    3. Depression
    4. Osteoporosis

Gonadal Hormones

chapter

38

Answer Key: Textbook page references are provided as a guide for answering these questions. A complete answer key is provided to your instructor.

MATCHING

Match the brand name drug on the right with the generic drug name on the left.

	Generic Drug Name		Brand Name Drug
1.	_____ esterified estrogen	a.	Aygestin
2.	_____ fluoxymesterone	b.	Estrace
3.	_____ conjugated estrogen	c.	Premarin
4.	_____ norethindrone	d.	Androxy
5.	_____ estradiol	e.	Methitest
6.	_____ methyltestosterone	f.	Menest

REVIEW QUESTIONS

Scenario: A 29-year-old male with hypogonadism comes into the clinic complaining of muscle cramps, tremors, and feeling tired. It was determined that he was experiencing an electrolyte imbalance from his medication.

Describe gonads and their function.

7. The ovaries produce estrogens that are responsible for the maturation of the uterus, as well as which characteristics evident at puberty? *(Select all that apply.)* *(589)*
   1. Nail growth
   2. Hair growth
   3. Muscle mass
   4. Skin texture
   5. Distribution of body fat
8. Estrogens have which effects on the body? *(Select all that apply.)* *(589)*
   1. They impact the release of gonadotropins.
   2. They cause fluid retention.
   3. They impact the release of gastrin in the stomach.
   4. They regulate protein metabolism.
   5. They cause elevated blood sugars.
9. What are androgens used to treat? *(Select all that apply.)* *(593)*
   1. Hypogonadism
   2. Severe acne
   3. Palliation of breast cancer
   4. Androgen deficiency
   5. Wasting syndrome associated with AIDS

Discuss the body changes that can be anticipated with the administration of androgens, estrogens, or progesterone.

10. When androgens are given to females, what effects can be anticipated? *(Select all that apply.)* *(593)*
    1. Gastric irritation
    2. Menstrual irregularity
    3. Electrolyte imbalance
    4. Deepening voice
    5. Clearing of acne
11. The nurse is teaching a patient about the adverse effects of estrogen therapy. Which statement by the patient indicates a need for further teaching? *(590)*
    1. "Weight gain is a common adverse effect of estrogen therapy."
    2. "Breast tenderness is to be expected when I start this drug."
    3. "Low blood pressure is a common side effect of estrogen therapy."
    4. "If I experience any breakthrough bleeding between my menstrual periods, I will notify my primary care provider immediately."
12. The nurse is teaching the patient in the scenario about ways to minimize the adverse effects of androgen therapy which include: *(Select all that apply.)* *(593)*
    1. drinking 8-12 glasses of water a day.

2. reporting any weight gain of more than 2 pounds per week.
3. including weight-bearing exercises in his ADLs.
4. chewing and swallowing the buccal tablet.
5. notifying the prescriber if nausea, anorexia, and jaundice occur.

13. The patient in the scenario is ordered testosterone USP in a gel base (Transdermal System) 5 mg every 24 hours. The nurse teaches the patient to rotate the application sites for the patch to which areas of the body? *(Select all that apply.)* *(594)*
    1. Hips
    2. Abdomen
    3. Thighs
    4. Buttocks
    5. Scrotum

Identify the uses of estrogens and progestins.

14. Progestin therapy is used to treat which conditions? *(Select all that apply.)* *(592)*
    1. Severe acne
    2. Breakthrough uterine bleeding
    3. Hot flash symptoms of menopause
    4. Endometriosis
    5. Secondary amenorrhea

15. The therapeutic uses for estrogen therapy are to: *(Select all that apply.)* *(589)*
    1. treat acne in males.
    2. relieve hot flash symptoms of menopause.
    3. treat advanced prostate cancer.
    4. treat osteoporosis.
    5. provide contraception.

16. When is the use of estrogens contraindicated? *(590)*
    1. With advanced prostatic cancer
    2. During early pregnancy
    3. During menopause
    4. Postpartum

Compare the adverse effects seen with the use of estrogen hormones with those seen with androgens.

17. While assessing a female patient on estrogen therapy for birth control, which adverse effect does the nurse report to the healthcare provider? *(590)*

1. Breakthrough bleeding
2. Weight gain
3. Breast tenderness
4. Nausea

18. Which gonadal hormone therapy is used for palliative treatment of prostate cancer? *(590)*
    1. Thyroid therapy
    2. Progestin therapy
    3. Androgen therapy
    4. Estrogen therapy

19. The nurse is teaching the patient in the scenario to report which effects of methyltestosterone to the healthcare provider? *(Select all that apply.)* *(593)*
    1. Masculinization
    2. Gastric irritation
    3. Weight gain of more than 2 pounds in a week
    4. Nausea, vomiting, constipation, and lethargy
    5. Jaundice, anorexia

20. When patients are started on estrogen therapy, which drug interactions may occur? *(Select all that apply.)* *(590)*
    1. Rifampin and estrogen may cause jaundice.
    2. Thyroid hormones and estrogens may cause hypothyroidism.
    3. Warfarin and estrogens may result in risk for clotting.
    4. Phenytoin and estrogens may cause toxicity of phenytoin.
    5. Insulin and estrogens may cause hypoglycemia.

21. Which serious adverse effects may be experienced with progestins? *(Select all that apply.)* *(592)*
    1. Cholestatic jaundice
    2. Depression
    3. Continuous headache
    4. Severe acne
    5. Weight gain and edema

Drugs Used in Obstetrics

Answer Key: Textbook page references are provided as a guide for answering these questions. A complete answer key is provided to your instructor.

MATCHING

Match the drug name on the right with the correct usage for the drug on the left.

Usage for Drug

1. _____ used to inhibit premature labor
2. _____ used to include labor at term
3. _____ used to expel uterine contents
4. _____ used to induce ovulation
5. _____ used as a cervical ripening agent
6. _____ used in small doses in postpartum patients to control bleeding

Drug

a. misoprostol
b. dinoprostone
c. methylergonovine maleate
d. oxytocin
e. magnesium sulfate
f. clomiphene citrate

REVIEW QUESTIONS

Scenario: A 32-year-old gravida 1, para 0, was admitted after 38 weeks gestation to the local delivery unit in possible labor. After the initial assessment, the patient was noted to have high blood pressure, pedal edema, and hyperreflexia. The patient was diagnosed with preeclampsia and was started on a magnesium sulfate infusion.

Identify appropriate nursing assessments during normal labor and delivery.

7. The nurse needs to be aware of which potential obstetric complications in pregnant women? *(Select all that apply.)* **(597)**
   1. Gestational diabetes
   2. Infection
   3. Preterm labor
   4. Hypoglycemia
   5. Premature rupture of membranes
8. The nurse was discussing postpartum care with a new mother and knew that more teaching was needed after the mother stated: **(604)**
   1. "I can take a mild analgesic 40 minutes before breastfeeding."
   2. "If I note any foul odor from my vaginal discharge, I know to call my healthcare provider."
   3. "I should use the breast pump prior to nursing my baby."

   4. "I know I need to continue to eat a well-balanced diet when breastfeeding."
9. Routine assessments performed on pregnant women no matter what trimester they are in include: *(Select all that apply.)* **(597)**
   1. weight.
   2. hemoglobin and hematocrit.
   3. blood pressure.
   4. vaginal exams.
   5. fundal height and fetal heart sounds.
10. Assessments of pregnant women include obtaining a history of: *(Select all that apply.)* **(597)**
    1. current medications.
    2. dietary practices.
    3. psychosocial and cultural patterns.
    4. previous obstetric history.
    5. sleep patterns.

Discuss potential complications of preterm labor and when uterine relaxants and magnesium sulfate are used.

11. The primary clinical indications for use of uterine stimulants include: *(Select all that apply.)* **(606)**
    1. induction or augmentation of labor.
    2. induction of therapeutic abortion.
    3. control of postpartum atony and hemorrhage.
    4. control of postsurgical hemorrhage.
    5. suppression of lactation.

12. What are some reasons for the use of uterine relaxants on the pregnant uterus? *(611)*
    1. They are used to suppress the flow of colostrum.
    2. They are used to delay or prevent labor and delivery in selected patients.
    3. They are used to induce or augment labor.
    4. They are used to control postpartum hemorrhage.
13. Which assessment findings that the nurse obtained from the patient in the scenario would indicate that the medication should be discontinued? *(612)*
    1. Absence of deep tendon reflexes
    2. Respiratory rate of 16 breaths/min
    3. Decrease in blood pressure from 180/100 to 150/90 mm Hg
    4. Urinary output of 45 mL during the past hour
14. What nursing action needs to be taken when pregnant women are in preterm labor? *(611)*
    1. Position the patient on her back.
    2. Administer uterine stimulants.
    3. Administer uterine relaxants.
    4. Restrict fluids.
15. What are signs of fetal distress? *(610)*
    1. Fetal heart rate >160 beats/min lasting less than 10 seconds after contractions
    2. Fetal heart rate 140 beats/min lasting longer than 15 seconds after contractions
    3. Fetal heart rate 120–160 beats/min following any contraction
    4. Fetal heart rate >160 followed by heart rate <120 occurring frequently following contractions

Describe when uterine stimulants are administered for induction of labor, augmentation of labor, and postpartum atony and hemorrhage.

16. The nurse assesses a patient receiving an infusion of oxytocin (Pitocin) to induce labor and determines the infant is in distress. Which actions does the nurse take? *(Select all that apply.)* *(610)*
    1. Turns the patient to the right lateral position
    2. Notifies the healthcare provider immediately
    3. Reduces the oxytocin infusion to the slowest possible rate according to hospital policy
    4. Administers oxygen by nasal cannula or facemask
    5. Administers a bolus of magnesium sulfate
17. The nurse was performing a postpartum assessment on a mother who was receiving oxytocin (Pitocin) therapy for control of bleeding and found the uterus to be boggy. What is the nurse's next action? *(611)*
    1. Administer magnesium sulfate.
    2. Slow the rate of the infusion.
    3. Call the healthcare provider immediately.
    4. Massage the uterus.
18. When working with patients receiving oxytocin (Pitocin), the nurse must assess for the development of water intoxication because oxytocin therapy causes which effect? *(610)*
    1. Extreme thirst in patients
    2. Hypocalcemia
    3. Stimulation of antidiuretic hormone
    4. Hypertension
19. List in correct order the steps to take for managing patients in preterm labor. *(599)*
    1. _____ Determine contraindications to tocolysis (i.e., placenta previa, fetal distress).
    2. _____ Monitor contractions and determine estimated gestational age.
    3. _____ Administer nifedipine and betamethasone.
    4. _____ Take vital signs of the mother and apply fetal monitoring.
    5. _____ Observe for cervical changes.
20. A patient is receiving magnesium sulfate to inhibit preterm labor. Which drug does the nurse have readily available if magnesium intoxication should occur? *(612)*
    1. Atropine
    2. Epinephrine
    3. Calcium gluconate
    4. Potassium chloride

State the actions of clomiphene citrate and the primary use.

21. Which drug is used to induce ovulation in women who are not ovulating because of low estrogen levels? *(613)*
    1. Magnesium sulfate
    2. Ergonovine maleate
    3. Clomiphene citrate
    4. Misoprostol
22. The nurse educates a woman who is taking clomiphene to get pregnant about precautions to take, including: *(Select all that apply.)* *(613)*
    1. "You need to take and record your temperature for one month after taking this."
    2. "If you do not get your period after a month you need to come back for a pregnancy test."
    3. "You need to take the medication every day for 5 days then wait to determine if ovulation occurs."
    4. "This medication may result in multiple fetuses."
    5. "Clomiphene usually takes three or four courses before it is effective."
23. A patient who is taking clomiphene to get pregnant asks the nurse about timing of intercourse. The best response by the nurse is: *(613)*
    1. "Timing does not matter; this medication will work no matter what you do."
    2. "You should time intercourse to occur when your temperature follows a biphasic pattern."
    3. "Intercourse should be timed during ovulation, usually 6 to 10 days after the last dose."

4. "It would be best to have intercourse at the same time every day for a month."

Identify the action and proper timing of the administration of Rho(D) immune globulin.

24. The recommended time of administration for Rho(D) immune globulin once the mother has delivered her baby is: *(614)*
    1. immediately after delivery.
    2. within 72 hours of delivery.
    3. only after the patient starts to hemorrhage.
    4. prior to discharge from the hospital.
25. What does Rho(D) immune globulin do when administered to patients? *(614)*
    1. It prevents Rh hemolytic disease in subsequent deliveries.
    2. It induces termination of pregnancy.
    3. It prevents postpartum gonorrhea infection.
    4. It prevents ovulation.
26. The nursing assessments needed prior to administration of Rho(D) immune globulin include checking: *(Select all that apply.)* *(614)*
    1. the Rh status of the mother.
    2. the platelet count of the mother.
    3. the Rh status of the infant.
    4. the platelet count of the infant.
    5. to determine if the mother is already sensitized.

Cite education needed for care of the neonate, including erythromycin ophthalmic ointment and phytonadione administration.

27. The health status of the neonate is estimated at 1 minute and 5 minutes after delivery using the Apgar rating system, which assesses which parameters of the newborn? *(Select all that apply.)* *(600)*

1. Heart rate
2. Blood pressure
3. Muscle tone
4. Reflex irritability
5. Color of body and extremities

28. Which procedures need to be attended to following the delivery of the newborn? *(Select all that apply.)* *(603-604)*
    1. Clamping the umbilical cord
    2. Airway—suction with bulb syringe if needed
    3. Eye prophylaxis
    4. Breastfeeding
    5. Determining an Apgar score
29. After birth all infants have prophylactic erythromycin ointment applied to their eyes to prevent: *(615)*
    1. pheochromocytoma.
    2. ophthalmia neonatorum.
    3. Wilms' tumor.
    4. nearsightedness.
30. A new mother asks the nurse why her newborn needs a shot of vitamin K. The nurse's response is: *(615)*
    1. "All babies get this to prevent ophthalmia neonatorum."
    2. "The delivery may have caused an infection in your baby and this will take care of it."
    3. "This will help increase the amount of natural bacteria in your baby's GI system."
    4. "Newborns are often deficient in vitamin K and we want to prevent any bleeding issues."

Drugs Used in Men's and Women's Health

Answer Key: Textbook page references are provided as a guide for answering these questions. A complete answer key is provided to your instructor.

MATCHING
Match the drug class on the right with the drug name on the left.

	Drug Name		Drug Class
1.	_____ Aranelle	a.	monophasic oral contraceptives
2.	_____ alfuzosin	b.	biphasic oral contraceptives
		c.	triphasic oral contraceptives
3.	_____ Alesse	d.	quadriphasic oral contraceptives
4.	_____ avanafil	e.	alpha-1 blocking agents
5.	_____ Natazia	f.	phosphodiesterase inhibitors
6.	_____ Amethia		

REVIEW QUESTIONS

Scenario: A couple came into the clinic with a request to be tested for gonorrhea and described abnormal vaginal discharge as well as urethral discharge from the penis.

Identify important personal hygiene measures to educate women and men regarding prevention of the spread of sexually transmitted infections.

7. Which patient education instructions are important to review when discussing hygiene measures with the couple in the scenario to prevent the spread of sexually transmitted infection? *(Select all that apply.)* *(621-622)*
   1. Urinate after intercourse.
   2. Douching after intercourse is effective in preventing pregnancy and HIV.
   3. Practice abstinence during the communicable phase of any disease.
   4. Spermicides, sponges, and diaphragms are effective in preventing transmission of HIV.
   5. Use latex condoms.
8. Which of these sexually transmitted infections are reportable by the health department in every state? *(Select all that apply.)* *(622)*
   1. Chlamydia
   2. Herpes simplex virus
   3. Syphilis
   4. Gonorrhea
   5. AIDS
9. The nurse is educating the couple in the scenario regarding preventing the spread of sexually transmitted infection and determines that further teaching is needed after hearing which comment? *(622)*
   1. The woman: "We will need to be abstinent from sex until this infection clears up."
   2. The man: "Next time, I can just use a condom."
   3. The woman: "I know I need to get a routine physical exam including a pelvic and breast exam and a Pap smear."
   4. The man: "I know I need to get a routine physical exam including a testicular exam, but not a rectal exam until I am over 40."
10. Hygiene measures are focused on educating the couple in the scenario on preventing: *(Select all that apply.)* *(621-622)*
    1. infections such as *Candida albicans* and *Trichomonas vaginalis*.
    2. secondary infections that may be acquired during the use of broad-spectrum antibiotics.
    3. development of endometriosis and uterine fibroids.
    4. unintended pregnancy.
    5. sexually transmitted infections.

Describe the major adverse effects and contraindications to the use of oral contraceptive agents.

11. Which adverse effect from the combination pill is of concern and needs to be reported as soon as possible? *(627)*
    1. Leg pain, chest pain, or shortness of breath
    2. Nausea
    3. Weight gain
    4. Chloasma

12. The minipill, which only contains progestin, is preferred by some women because of their history of which conditions that are aggravated by estrogens? *(Select all that apply.) (625)*
    1. Migraines
    2. Hypertension
    3. Hypothyroidism
    4. Depression
    5. Diabetes

13. Why is smoking while on the pill considered to be so risky for women? *(625)*
    1. The chance of pregnancy is increased.
    2. The possibility of breakthrough bleeding is increased.
    3. The pill loses its effectiveness after just one cigarette.
    4. The likelihood of developing a serious blood clot is increased.

14. Which type of combination pill is used for patients who have heavy menses with associated anemia? *(625)*
    1. Biphasic
    2. Triphasic
    3. Continuous cycle
    4. Monophasic

15. What precaution must be taken prior to starting birth control pills? *(625)*
    1. Determine if any sexually transmitted infections have been contracted.
    2. Ensure that the patient is not pregnant.
    3. Obtain a list of past sexual partners.
    4. Determine the sperm count of the male partner.

16. How does the combination pill produce contraception differently from the minipill? *(623)*
    1. By causing the cervical mucus to become thicker
    2. By inhibiting the release of luteinizing hormone
    3. By causing sperm migration to be inhibited by viscous mucus
    4. By blocking the pituitary release of follicle-stimulating hormone

Identify the patient teaching necessary with the administration of the transdermal contraceptive and the intravaginal hormonal contraceptive.

17. In teaching a patient about the use of norelgestromin-ethinyl estradiol transdermal system (Ortho Evra), which statements does the nurse include? *(Select all that apply.) (628)*

1. "Trim the patch to best fit the area where you wish to apply it."
2. "Do not place the patch on your breast."
3. "Avoid lotions or creams on the areas of the skin where the patch is applied because the patch may not adhere properly."
4. "If the patch is partially detached for less than 24 hours, try to reapply it in the same place or replace it with a new patch immediately."
5. "Apply the patch to the buttock, abdomen, upper outer arm, or upper torso."

18. What serious adverse effects must be reported with the use of the NuvaRing? *(Select all that apply.) (630)*
    1. Vaginal discharge and yeast infection
    2. Breakthrough bleeding
    3. Constipation
    4. Blurred vision and severe headaches
    5. Leg pain, chest pain, shortness of breath

19. Which information does the nurse include when teaching a patient about the use of the norelgestromin-ethinyl estradiol transdermal system (Ortho Evra)? *(Select all that apply.) (628)*
    1. "A new patch should be applied on the same day of the week."
    2. "Apply the first patch during the first 24 hours of the menstrual period or on the first Sunday after menses begin."
    3. "If the patch is detached for less than 24 hours, apply a new patch to the same location."
    4. "If two consecutive periods are missed, a pregnancy test is in order."
    5. "Contraceptive therapy should be discontinued if pregnancy is confirmed."

Describe pharmacologic treatments of benign prostatic hyperplasia.

20. A nurse is describing the difference between the symptoms of obstructive and irritative benign prostatic hyperplasia (BPH) to a patient. Which statement needs to be amended? *(631)*
    1. "The symptoms of irritative BPH include having a decreased or interrupted urine stream."
    2. "The symptoms of obstructive BPH include having a reduced urine flow."
    3. "The symptoms of irritative BPH include having sudden urinary urgency."
    4. "The symptoms of obstructive BPH include having the sensation of incomplete bladder emptying."

21. When teaching a patient about dutasteride (Avodart) therapy for BPH, which statement does the nurse include? *(633)*
    1. "If there is no improvement of symptoms after 2 weeks of treatment, the dutasteride will be discontinued."
    2. "Men treated with dutasteride should not donate blood until at least 6 months after stopping therapy."

3. "Dutasteride is used to treat male pattern baldness."
4. "Dutasteride will cause an increase in serum prostate-specific antigen (PSA) levels."
22. Which medications used for BPH work by inhibiting 5-alpha reductase type 2? *(Select all that apply.)* *(633)*
   1. Finasteride
   2. Tamsulosin
   3. Dutasteride
   4. Sildenafil
   5. Silodosin

Describe the pharmacologic treatment of erectile dysfunction.

23. The nurse is teaching a patient about tadalafil (Cialis) therapy. Which statement made by the patient indicates teaching has been successful? *(635)*
   1. "This drug is an aphrodisiac."
   2. "I will take this medication three times a day on a regular basis."
   3. "I can expect the medication to work within 30 minutes."
   4. "If I develop chest pain, I will take nitroglycerin."
24. Which classification of drugs is used to treat erectile dysfunction? *(634)*
   1. Androgen hormone inhibitors
   2. Phosphodiesterase inhibitors
   3. Alpha-1 adrenergic blockers
   4. Butyrophenones

25. Which statement made by the patient about sildenafil (Viagra) therapy indicates further teaching is needed? *(636)*
   1. "I know that I should not take nitroglycerin for any angina while I am on Viagra."
   2. "I understand that if I suddenly lose my vision I need to report it immediately."
   3. "If I get an erection that lasts longer than 4 hours I will seek medical attention."
   4. "I know that Viagra can cause patients to develop glaucoma."
26. The nurse is educating the patient on the common adverse effects to expect when taking avanafil (Stendra) to treat erectile dysfunction, and includes: *(Select all that apply.)* *(636)*
   1. "If you develop any headache or flushing in your face and neck, these symptoms tend to be self-limiting."
   2. "It has been reported that if you become colorblind to blue or green, call your prescriber to get a dosage adjustment."
   3. "If you get dizzy or develop low blood pressure, lie down and let the symptoms pass."
   4. "Call your prescriber right away if you develop a sudden loss of vision."
   5. "You need to be careful with nitrates in your foods as they will react with the avanafil."

Drugs Used to Treat Disorders of the Urinary System

chapter **41**

Answer Key: Textbook page references are provided as a guide for answering these questions. A complete answer key is provided to your instructor.

MATCHING

Match the definition on the right with the key term on the left.

Key Term		Definition
1. _____ acidification	a.	the need to void eight or more times daily
2. _____ pyelonephritis	b.	waking during the night with the need to void
3. _____ frequency	c.	the need to urinate frequently both day and night
4. _____ urgency	d.	administering vitamin C to lower the pH of the urine
5. _____ overactive bladder syndrome	e.	infection of the kidney
	f.	a compelling desire to urinate that is difficult to ignore
6. _____ nocturia	g.	the inability to control urine from passing from the bladder
7. _____ incontinence		

REVIEW QUESTIONS

Scenario: A 52-year-old female patient came to the clinic with complaints of burning on urination and foul-smelling urine. She told the nurse that this happens about twice a year.

Explain the major actions of drugs used to treat disorders of the urinary tract.

8. Which conditions are examples of common urinary tract infections? *(Select all that apply.)* **(638)**
    1. Vaginitis
    2. Cystitis
    3. Pyelonephritis
    4. Urethritis
    5. Prostatitis
9. Which antimicrobial agents are used for bladder infections? *(Select all that apply.)* **(641)**
    1. Linezolid
    2. Fosfomycin
    3. Azithromycin
    4. Norfloxacin
    5. Nitrofurantoin
10. Which statements about phenazopyridine hydrochloride (Pyridium) for the treatment of patients with urinary tract infections are correct? *(Select all that apply.)* **(647)**

1. Pyridium produces a local anesthetic effect on the mucosa of the ureters and bladder.
2. Pyridium is most effective against gram-negative bacterial urinary tract infections.
3. Pyridium relieves burning, pain, urgency, and frequency associated with urinary tract infections.
4. Pyridium reduces bladder spasms.
5. Pyridium causes the color of urine to become reddish-orange.

11. A postpartum patient who had a complicated vaginal delivery of a baby 9 hours ago is unable to void despite multiple nonpharmacologic interventions by the nurse. The nurse expects the healthcare provider to order which drug to facilitate bladder tone and urination? **(645)**
    1. Bethanechol chloride (Urecholine)
    2. Neostigmine (Prostigmin)
    3. Oxybutynin chloride (Ditropan)
    4. Tolterodine (Detrol)
12. What is often prescribed to help maintain the acidity of the urine? **(642)**
    1. Vitamin A
    2. *Ginkgo biloba*
    3. Vitamin C
    4. St. John's wort

13. Which drug acts by interfering with several bacterial enzyme systems? *(643)*
    1. Cinoxacin
    2. Norfloxacin
    3. Nalidixic acid
    4. Nitrofurantoin

Identify baseline data that the nurse should collect for comparison and evaluation of drug effectiveness.

14. The nurse will gather what baseline data from the patient in the scenario? *(Select all that apply.)* *(639)*
    1. Reviews the laboratory results for the organism causing the infection
    2. Seeks cooperation and understanding of the medication regimen
    3. Assesses the symptoms of urinary frequency, pain, and any retention
    4. Obtains a urinalysis
    5. Follows up on adherence with the therapy prescribed

15. An important assessment needed to determine the effectiveness of antimicrobial agents for urinary infections is: *(641)*
    1. determine the degree of stress incontinence.
    2. a follow-up culture to be collected to assess success of the therapy.
    3. determine if the adverse effect of vision disturbance has occurred.
    4. verify the instructions for acidification of the urine.

16. Which antimicrobial agent has been approved as a single-dose treatment for urinary tract infections? *(642)*
    1. Nitrofurantoin
    2. Methenamine mandelate
    3. Fosfomycin
    4. Nalidixic acid

Identify important nursing implementations associated with the drug therapy and treatment of diseases of the urinary system.

17. Which patients are considered to have a urinary tract infection? *(Select all that apply.)* *(638)*
    1. Male with pyelonephritis
    2. Female diagnosed with cystitis
    3. Male with prostatitis
    4. 4-year-old male with urethritis
    5. Female with vaginitis

18. A patient is experiencing burning, frequency, pain, and urgency associated with a urinary tract infection. The nurse expects the healthcare provider to order which medication to treat these symptoms? *(647)*
    1. Phenazopyridine hydrochloride (Pyridium)
    2. Oxybutynin chloride (Ditropan)
    3. Methenamine mandelate (Mandelamine)
    4. Nitrofurantoin (Macrodantin)

19. The nurse knows that an important component of patient education to enhance compliance with medications is to determine if the patient can verbalize: *(Select all that apply.)* *(641)*
    1. identification of the specific pathogen.
    2. name of drug.
    3. common and adverse effects of the drug.
    4. dosage of the drug.
    5. time of administration of the drug.

20. What important health teaching should the nurse complete for the patient in the scenario? *(Select all that apply.)* *(641)*
    1. Drink plenty of fluids—2000 mL or more per day.
    2. Return for urine culture when scheduled.
    3. Discuss personal hygiene measures—wiping front to back in females, keeping perineal area clean.
    4. Continue the medication for the entire course of treatment.
    5. If symptoms such as perineal itching or vaginal discharge occur, wait several days to see if they will resolve on their own.

Identify the symptoms, treatment, and medication used for overactive bladder syndrome.

21. Which statements does the nurse include when teaching a patient about overactive bladder syndrome? *(Select all that apply.)* *(644)*
    1. "The first line of pharmacologic treatment of overactive bladder syndrome is the anticholinergic agents."
    2. "Overactive bladder syndrome cannot be cured."
    3. "You should avoid caffeine."
    4. "The goals of therapy for overactive bladder syndrome are to decrease frequency by increasing voided volume, decreasing urgency, and reducing incidents of urinary urge incontinence."
    5. "A chronic infection is the cause of overactive bladder syndrome."

22. Which drugs are included in anticholinergic agents used for overactive bladder syndrome? *(Select all that apply.)* *(646)*
    1. Darifenacin
    2. Norfloxacin
    3. Neostigmine
    4. Oxybutynin
    5. Trospium

23. What are the three primary symptoms of overactive bladder syndrome? *(644)*
    1. Frequency, urinary infections, urinary incontinence
    2. Urgency, nocturia, urge incontinence
    3. Nocturia, frequency, stress incontinence
    4. Frequency, urgency, and urinary incontinence

24. Which statements made by the nurse when teaching the patient in the scenario about methenamine mandelate (Mandelamine) are correct? *(Select all that apply.)* **(642)**
    1. "The tablets should not be crushed, as this will allow the formation of formaldehyde in the stomach."
    2. This drug should be administered with sodium bicarbonate."
    3. "Careful when taking this with vitamin C as it will become inactive."
    4. "You should not discontinue taking this drug if nausea, vomiting, and belching develop without first consulting your healthcare provider."
    5. "This drug is used for patients like you who have chronic, recurrent urinary tract infections."

25. The nurse is teaching the patient in the scenario about measures that can be taken to prevent the recurrence of urinary tract infections, including: *(Select all that apply.)* **(640)**
    1. "It is recommended that you take frequent bubble baths and wear tight underwear."
    2. "When you are on these medications for your infection, you will need to drink plenty of fluids."
    3. "You only have to take these drugs until your symptoms clear up."
    4. "It is best to take your antimicrobial agent exactly as prescribed for the entire course of the medication."
    5. "You need to maintain adequate urine volume as a means to treat the overall problem of having recurrent urinary tract infections."

Drugs Used to Treat Glaucoma and Other Eye Disorders

Answer Key: Textbook page references are provided as a guide for answering these questions. A complete answer key is provided to your instructor.

MATCHING
Match the key term on the right with the definition on the left.

	Definition		Key Term
1. _____	runs radially from the pupillary margin to the iris periphery	a.	miosis
2. _____	sudden increase in IOP caused by an obstruction in the iridocorneal angle	b.	mydriasis
		c.	cycloplegia
3. _____	dilation of the pupils	d.	sphincter muscle
4. _____	within the iris that encircles the pupil	e.	open-angle glaucoma
5. _____	paralysis of the ciliary muscle	f.	closed-angle glaucoma
6. _____	contraction of the iris sphincter muscle	g.	dilator muscle
7. _____	develops insidiously and causes changes in the iridocorneal angle		

REVIEW QUESTIONS

Scenario: A 63-year-old male patient comes into the clinic with complaints of pain and constant tearing in his right eye after a flag whipped around his head and caught his eye. He is diagnosed with a corneal abrasion.

Describe the anatomy and physiology of the eye and the normal flow of aqueous humor.

8. What are the layers of the eye? *(Select all that apply.)* *(649)*
   1. Zonular fibers
   2. Choroid
   3. Retina
   4. Corneoscleral coat
   5. Aqueous humor
9. The nurse was educating the patient in the scenario on the anatomy and physiology of the eye. Which statements would be included in the discussion? *(Select all that apply.)* *(649)*
   1. "The pupil, or the hole in the iris, is the center black portion of the eye that allows light to reach the retina."
   2. "The cornea is the outermost sheath of the anterior eyeball and is transparent."
   3. "The lens is a transparent, gelatinous mass of fibers encased in an elastic capsule situated behind the iris."
   4. "When the cornea becomes abraded, it is highly susceptible to infection."
   5. "The aqueous humor secretes tears that wash away foreign objects from the eye."
10. The term *mydriasis* is defined as the: *(649)*
    1. paralysis of the ciliary muscle.
    2. contraction of the dilator muscle and relaxation of the sphincter muscle, which cause the pupil to dilate.
    3. contraction of the iris sphincter muscle, which causes the pupil to narrow.
    4. drainage of aqueous humor out of the eye through drainage channels.
11. How does the eye receive nutrients? *(649)*
    1. Through the aqueous humor
    2. Through the blood vessels
    3. Through the thin layer of epithelial cells on the surface of the cornea
    4. Through the sclera, or the white portion of the eye

12. List in order the flow of aqueous humor in the eye. *(650)*

    1. _____ Flows forward between the lens and the iris into the anterior chamber.
    2. _____ The ciliary body secretes aqueous humor.
    3. _____ Drains out of the eye through drainage channels located near the junction of the cornea and sclera into a meshwork that leads into Schlemm's canal.
    4. _____ It bathes and feeds the lens, the posterior surface of the cornea, and iris.
    5. _____ It flows into the venous system of the eye.

13. When patients have their intraocular pressure (IOP) measured, it determines the eye's: *(651)*
    1. tear duct capacity.
    2. resistance from the ciliary bodies.
    3. amount of aqueous humor.
    4. ability to contract and relax the dilator muscle.

Identify the changes in normal flow of aqueous humor caused by open-angle and closed-angle glaucoma.

14. What happens when patients have open-angle glaucoma? *(651)*
    1. The sudden increase in IOP is caused by a mechanical obstruction in the iridocorneal angle.
    2. IOP is gradually increased because of the changes in the iridocorneal angle that prevent the outflow of aqueous humor.
    3. The posterior chamber narrows, causing an increase in IOP.
    4. The anterior chamber overflows into the posterior chamber, causing an increase in IOP.

15. The nurse was discussing the difference between open-angle glaucoma and closed-angle glaucoma with a patient who was newly diagnosed with glaucoma. Which statement by the patient indicates more teaching is needed? *(652)*
    1. "Closed-angle glaucoma is the one that suddenly develops."
    2. "Open-angle glaucoma is the kind that develops slowly."
    3. "Glaucoma is an eye disorder that develops because the pressure inside your eyeball is too high."
    4. "Glaucoma can be cured by taking eyedrops for 2 weeks."

16. Of the three types of glaucoma, which one requires surgical intervention to correct? *(652)*
    1. Primary
    2. Secondary
    3. Tertiary
    4. Congenital

Explain patient assessments needed for eye disorders.

17. What is typically included in an eye exam that the nurse performs for the patient in the scenario with an eye injury? *(Select all that apply.)* *(652)*
    1. Check for edema.
    2. Observe for any redness or drainage of the eyes.
    3. Ask whether there is any history of colorblindness.
    4. Observe for and report nystagmus.
    5. Ask whether glasses or contact lenses are worn.

18. One of the greatest challenges in the care of chronic eye disorders such as glaucoma is convincing the patient of the: *(652)*
    1. importance of not taking any over-the-counter or herbal products.
    2. differences among cataracts, glaucoma, and macular degeneration.
    3. need for long-term treatment and adherence to the therapeutic regimen.
    4. need to wear an eye patch every night to prevent eye strain.

19. What adverse effects will the nurse assess for in patients who are receiving cholinergic agents that produce strong contractions of the iris, which widen the filtration angle? *(656)*
    1. Circulatory overload symptoms
    2. Diminished visual acuity checks
    3. Allergies to sulfonamide antibiotics
    4. Bleeding tendencies

Review the correct procedure for instilling eyedrops or eye ointments and discuss patient teaching needs for glaucoma medication use.

20. List in the correct order how to instill eyedrops or eye ointment. *(654)*
    1. _____ Perform hand hygiene and don gloves.
    2. _____ Approach the eye from below.
    3. _____ Apply gentle pressure using a clean tissue to the inner canthus of the eyelid.
    4. _____ Instruct the patient to look up, and instill drops or squeeze ointment into the conjunctival sac.
    5. _____ Expose the lower conjunctival sac by applying gentle traction.

21. Which statements does the nurse include when teaching a patient about health promotion after eye surgery? *(Select all that apply.)* *(654)*
    1. "Avoid bending at the waist."
    2. "Avoid any straining with stool."
    3. "Report any pain not relieved by prescribed medications."
    4. "Use aseptic technique when instilling eye medications."
    5. "Cough at least 10 times every hour."

22. To prevent systemic effects of ophthalmic cholinergic agents, the nurse carefully blocks the inner canthus of the eye for how many minutes? *(657)*
    1. 1–2
    2. 3–5
    3. 8–10
    4. 12–14
23. What are systemic adverse effects of the anticholinergic agent atropine sulfate (Isopto-Atropine)? *(Select all that apply.)* *(661)*
    1. Bradycardia
    2. Diarrhea
    3. Blurred vision
    4. Vasodilation
    5. Dry mouth
24. What mechanism of action do carbonic anhydrase inhibitors have on the eye? *(655)*
    1. They inhibit the enzyme carbonic anhydrase, which results in a decrease in aqueous humor production.
    2. They decrease the flow of aqueous humor by closing the iridocorneal angle.
    3. They widen the filtration angle, permitting an outflow of aqueous humor.
    4. They increase tearing and widen the nasolacrimal ducts.
25. Cholinergic agents produce contraction of the iris (miosis) and ciliary body musculature (accommodation), by which mechanism of action? *(656)*
    1. They absorb acetylcholine at nerve synapses.
    2. They cause vasoconstriction of the blood vessels in the eye.

3. Their effect results in a reduced production of aqueous humor.
4. They cause a widening of the filtration angle, thus decreasing IOP.
26. Adrenergic agents have several mechanisms of action, including: *(Select all that apply.)* *(657)*
    1. causing pupil dilation and relaxation of ciliary muscle.
    2. causing a decrease in the formation of aqueous humor.
    3. causing an increase in the outflow of aqueous humor.
    4. causing vasoconstriction of the blood vessels in the eye.
    5. absorbing an excess volume of aqueous humor.
27. How are beta-adrenergic blocking agents thought to work when given for the treatment of glaucoma? *(658)*
    1. Increasing the filtration angle, thus decreasing IOP
    2. Reducing production of aqueous humor
    3. Absorbing the excess volume of aqueous humor
    4. Inhibiting any cholinergic activity within the eye
28. What mechanism of action do prostaglandin agonists have on the eye? *(659)*
    1. They absorb aqueous humor.
    2. They reduce IOP by increasing the outflow of aqueous humor.
    3. They cause vasoconstriction of the blood vessels in the eye.
    4. They reduce the production of aqueous humor.

Drugs Used to Treat Cancer

chapter

43

Answer Key: Textbook page references are provided as a guide for answering these questions. A complete answer key is provided to your instructor.

MATCHING

Match the chemotherapeutic agent on the right with its classification on the left.

Chemotherapeutic Classification

1. _____ alkylating agents
2. _____ antimetabolites
3. _____ natural products
4. _____ antineoplastic antibodies
5. _____ hormones
6. _____ biologic therapies

Chemotherapeutic Agent

a. dactinomycin
b. vascular endothelial growth factor
c. methotrexate
d. paclitaxel
e. cisplatin
f. tamoxifen

REVIEW QUESTIONS

Scenario: A 48-year-old woman, mother of three, was newly diagnosed with breast cancer and was very distraught in the outpatient clinic when she came for her first chemotherapy treatment.

Cite the goals of chemotherapy.

7. Which are goals of chemotherapy? *(Select all that apply.)* *(668)*
    1. Give doses large enough to kill the cancer cells but small enough for normal cells to live.
    2. Control growth of the cancer cells.
    3. Long-term survival or a cure of cancer.
    4. Give when new pathways of tumor cell metabolism are discovered.
    5. Use phase-nonspecific chemotherapy agents exclusively.
8. After educating the patient in the scenario about the best timing for giving chemotherapy, the nurse knows that which statement by the patient would indicate further teaching is needed? *(675)*
    1. "I know that the overall goal of chemotherapy in general is to give enough drug to kill the cancer without too much damage to the normal cells."
    2. "I understand it is important to deliver the chemotherapy at precise intervals to impact the cancer cells' growth cycle."

3. "If I am proactive about preventing side effects from the chemotherapy, I can learn to manage my symptoms."
4. "I understand that when I am on chemotherapy, I can determine how often I have to have it depending on my symptoms."

9. For the patient and family to manage the chemotherapy treatment regimen, an understanding of which points needs to be stressed? *(Select all that apply.)* *(675)*
    1. Name of the drug
    2. Right indication
    3. Common and serious adverse effects
    4. Time of administration
    5. Dosage and route of the drug
10. Treatment of cancer often requires multiple different approaches, which may include: *(Select all that apply.)* *(667)*
    1. surgery.
    2. radiation.
    3. biologic therapies.
    4. targeted drug therapy.
    5. phlebotomy.

Describe the role of targeted anticancer agents in treating cancer.

11. The choice of chemotherapeutic agents used to help fight cancer depends on the: *(Select all that apply.)* *(669)*
    1. size of the tumor.

2.　frequency of the agents' administration.

3.　rate of growth of the cancer.

4.　type of tumor cell.

5.　potency of the agent.

12.　What is the role of targeted anticancer agents in treating cancer? *(669)*

1.　They reduce the toxic effects of the chemotherapy agents.

2.　They cause cell death by means that are unknown.

3.　They trigger the recovery of the bone marrow cells.

4.　They act on receptors that are specific to the cancer cells' growth factors.

13.　Which are considered part of the traditional major groups of chemotherapeutic agents? *(Select all that apply.)* *(669)*

1.　Antimetabolites

2.　Natural products

3.　Prostaglandin inhibitors

4.　Hormones

5.　Antineoplastic antibiotics

14.　Biologic therapies or targeted anticancer agents include: *(Select all that apply.)* *(669)*

1.　cholinesterase inhibitors.

2.　growth factors.

3.　vaccines.

4.　monoclonal antibodies.

5.　cytokines.

Identify how chemoprotective agents are used in treating cancer.

15.　The reason chemoprotective agents are used to treat cancer is because they: *(670)*

1.　reduce the toxic effects of the chemotherapy agents on normal cells.

2.　target the cancer cells specifically.

3.　trigger the recovery of bone marrow cells.

4.　stimulate red blood cell production.

16.　Which medications are used as chemoprotective agents? *(Select all that apply.)* *(670)*

1.　Sargramostim (Leukine)

2.　Mesna (Mesnex)

3.　Dexrazoxane (Zinecard)

4.　Amifostine (Ethyol)

5.　Vorinostat (Zolinza)

17.　The nurse was explaining to the patient in the scenario the reason for the medication Totect that she was receiving after her chemotherapy. Which statement by the patient indicates further teaching is needed? *(670)*

1.　"I understand that Totect is to reduce the chances of developing cardiomyopathy from the doxorubicin I'm taking."

2.　"The drug Totect will stimulate my bone marrow to produce red blood cells."

3.　"Because I am taking Totect, I know that I will not get as sick from my chemotherapy."

4.　"As I understand it, this drug Totect is designed to reduce the toxic effects of my chemotherapy."

18.　The nurse is administering a chemotherapeutic agent and knows precautions must be observed for safe handling such as: *(Select all that apply.)* *(670)*

1.　preventing any inhalation of aerosols.

2.　carefully mixing the agents in the med room.

3.　preventing contamination of body fluids.

4.　expecting that the dosage of the agents depends on the cancer.

5.　preventing any drug absorption through the skin.

Discuss bone marrow stimulants and their effect and use.

19.　What do the bone marrow stimulants do in the treatment of cancer? *(670)*

1.　They stimulate the resting phase of the cell.

2.　They trigger an increase of killer T cells.

3.　They trigger the recovery of bone marrow cells.

4.　They induce anemia.

20.　The nurse anticipates the use of which medication to treat a patient with chemotherapy-induced anemia? *(671)*

1.　Sargramostim (Leukine)

2.　Oprelvekin (Neumega)

3.　Filgrastim (Neupogen)

4.　Epoetin alfa (Epogen)

21.　In which situation would the use of bone marrow stimulants be appropriate? *(Select all that apply.)* *(670)*

1.　When treating leukemia.

2.　During bone marrow transplantation.

3.　To control cell membrane receptor response.

4.　To reduce the toxic effects of chemotherapy.

5.　During lymphoma therapy.

22.　Use of bone marrow stimulants to allow the immune system to recover earlier than would occur naturally results in the major benefit of: *(670)*

1.　allowing the patient to have fewer cycles of chemotherapy.

2.　stopping infections from becoming pathologic.

3.　preventing chronic renal failure.

4.　delaying the effects of anticipated nausea and vomiting.

Describe the nursing assessments and interventions needed to help alleviate the adverse effects of chemotherapy.

23.　The baseline assessments by the nurse for the patient in the scenario needed during the initiation of cancer therapy include: *(Select all that apply.)* *(672)*

1.　the emotional status of the patient.

2.　the family's expectation of therapy.

3.　the understanding the patient has of the diagnosis.

4.　the patient's usual methods of coping.

5.　usual eating and elimination patterns.

24. Which adverse effects from chemotherapy does the nurse monitor patients for? *(Select all that apply.)* *(673)*
    1. Stomatitis
    2. Changes in bowel patterns
    3. Infection
    4. Nausea and vomiting
    5. Heat intolerance
25. A patient has severe lesions in his mouth as an adverse effect of chemotherapy. When does the nurse suggest the patient perform oral hygiene measures using prescribed local anesthetic and antimicrobial solutions? *(673)*

    1. In the morning when the patient awakens and before bed.
    2. After each meal.
    3. Once every 8 hours.
    4. Hourly while the patient is awake.
26. Cancer care that applies to all patients includes: *(Select all that apply.)* *(672)*
    1. anticipating that diarrhea will occur.
    2. determining activity tolerance.
    3. allowing rest periods.
    4. attending to pain management.
    5. limiting the amount of self-care allowed.

Drugs Used to Treat the Musculoskeletal System

Answer Key: Textbook page references are provided as a guide for answering these questions. A complete answer key is provided to your instructor.

MATCHING
Match the definition on the left to the key term on the right.

Key Term

1. _____ cerebral palsy
2. _____ multiple sclerosis
3. _____ stroke syndrome
4. _____ hypercapnia
5. _____ spasticity
6. _____ muscle spasms

Definition

a. an upper motor neuron disorder characterized by muscle hypertonicity and involuntary jerks
b. caused by an injury or birth defect, characterized by exaggerated reflexes, abnormal posture, involuntary movements, and difficulty walking
c. elevated carbon dioxide levels causing tachycardia, hypotension, and cyanosis
d. sudden alternating contractions and relaxations or sustained contractions of muscle
e. an autoimmune disease affecting the brain and spinal cord
f. caused by an embolism, thrombosis, or ruptured aneurysm; characteristics include a sudden onset of vertigo, numbness, aphasia, and dysarthria, along with hemiplegia

REVIEW QUESTIONS

Scenario: A 35-year-old male patient with cerebral palsy came into the outpatient clinic because he was scheduled to have his baclofen pump refilled.

Describe the nursing assessment data needed to evaluate a patient with a skeletal muscle disorder.

7. The nurse will need to obtain a medication history from the patient in the scenario, and asks: *(Select all that apply.)* **(679)**
   1. "What is the extent of your usual daily exercise?"
   2. "What medications did you take today and when?"
   3. "Do you use any nonpharmacologic treatments like a heating pad or acupuncture?"
   4. "Do you use any assistive devices?"
   5. "Do you have a list of all the prescribed and over-the-counter medications that you are taking?"
8. A 32-year-old man came to the outpatient clinic complaining about a recent injury sustained while jogging and subsequent left knee pain. The nurse knows further education is needed after the patient states: **(680)**
   1. "I can put ice on my knee to help with the swelling for 48 hours."
   2. "I will have to elevate my leg initially to reduce swelling and pain."
   3. "I can immobilize my knee with an elastic wrap to help with the pain."
   4. "I can use hot packs on my knee initially to help with the pain."
9. The nurse needs to gather important assessment data on the patient in the scenario including: *(Select all that apply.)* **(679)**
   1. noting any differences in circumference, symmetry, or length of limbs.
   2. evaluating the capillary refill and any presence of paresthesias.
   3. assessing mental status.
   4. assessing muscle strength by asking the patient to lift his head off the pillow.
   5. determining the degree of respiratory depression.

Identify the therapeutic response and the common and serious adverse effects from skeletal muscle relaxant therapy.

10. What is the mechanism of action for the centrally acting skeletal muscle relaxants? **(681)**

1. They directly affect the muscles.
2. They cause CNS depression.
3. They affect nerve conduction.
4. They cause the neuromuscular junctions to be desensitized to stimuli.

11. Which statement by a patient taking dantrolene (Dantrium) for treatment of muscle spasticity of stroke syndrome indicates that more patient education is needed? *(684)*
    1. "I will avoid exposure to the sun, but I can still use a tanning lamp."
    2. "If I develop adverse effects from this medication, I will not discontinue treatment until I notify my healthcare provider."
    3. "I will notify my healthcare provider if my skin turns yellow."
    4. "I know that it might take up to a week for me to see any response to this drug."

12. For which adverse effects does the nurse need to evaluate the patient in the scenario, related to the baclofen pump? *(Select all that apply.)* *(683)*
    1. Drowsiness
    2. Fatigue
    3. Headache
    4. Back pain
    5. Dizziness

Describe the effect of centrally acting skeletal muscle relaxants on the central nervous system (CNS) and the safety precautions required during their use.

13. Which statements about centrally acting skeletal muscle relaxants are true? *(Select all that apply.)* *(681)*
    1. They directly relax the muscles by suppressing nerve conduction at the neuromuscular junction.
    2. They produce sedation in patients receiving them.
    3. They are the agents of choice for the treatment of muscle spasticity associated with cerebral or spinal cord disease.
    4. They produce their therapeutic effect by depressing the central nervous system.
    5. They have a direct effect on the neuromuscular junction, causing relaxation.

14. The nurse was reviewing which laboratory results to determine if the patient on chlorzoxazone (Lorzone) was exhibiting any hepatotoxicity? *(Select all that apply.)* *(682)*
    1. GGT
    2. WBC
    3. RBC
    4. AST
    5. ALT

15. Which medications are considered centrally acting skeletal muscle relaxants? *(Select all that apply.)* *(682)*
    1. Metaxalone (Skelaxin)
    2. Dantrolene (Dantrium)

3. Cyclobenzaprine (Flexeril)
4. Vecuronium
5. Carisoprodol (Soma)

Describe the physiologic effects of neuromuscular blocking agents and assessments needed, as well as the equipment needed in the immediate patient care area when neuromuscular blocking agents are administered.

16. Which are examples of when it would be appropriate to use neuromuscular blocking agents? *(Select all that apply.)* *(684)*
    1. When patients have tetanus.
    2. During the administration of electroshock therapy to prevent muscular activity.
    3. When intubating patients and preventing laryngospasm.
    4. When patients develop nystagmus.
    5. During the administration of general anesthesia.

17. Why would patients with myasthenia gravis, spinal cord injuries, or multiple sclerosis need to be carefully identified prior to administration of neuromuscular blocking agents? *(684)*
    1. They will develop the adverse effect of histamine release much faster than other patients.
    2. They will require larger doses of the agents to get the same effect as other patients.
    3. They need careful adjustments in dosages because of the insensitivity of their neuromuscular junctions.
    4. Postoperatively, they will experience respiratory depression for a prolonged period.

18. Which drugs are antidotes for neuromuscular blocking agents? *(Select all that apply.)* *(684)*
    1. Edrophonium chloride (Enlon)
    2. Pyridostigmine bromide (Mestinon)
    3. Naloxone (Narcan)
    4. Neostigmine methylsulfate (Prostigmin)
    5. Propranolol hydrochloride (Inderal)

19. A patient who has returned from abdominal surgery reports pain. The patient had received a neuromuscular blocking agent as part of the anesthesia for the surgery. What additional information is essential for the nurse to obtain before administering the prescribed analgesic? *(685)*
    1. Laboratory results for CBC and electrolytes
    2. Vital signs
    3. Family history
    4. Estimated time of discharge

20. Which description of patients receiving neuromuscular blocking agents is accurate? *(685)*
    1. They are at risk for the development of bronchospasm, edema, and urticaria.
    2. They experience complete analgesia.
    3. They have an enhanced cough reflex.
    4. They experience a decrease in salivation.

21. Which statements about the effects of neuromuscular blocking agents in patients with muscular disorders are true? *(Select all that apply.)* **(684)**
    1. Neuromuscular blocking agents have no effect on consciousness.
    2. Neuromuscular blocking agents have no effect on memory.
    3. Neuromuscular blocking agents have no effect on pain threshold.
    4. Pain medications are contraindicated in patients receiving neuromuscular blocking agents.
    5. The IV route is the only method for administering neuromuscular blocking agents.

Antimicrobial Agents

Answer Key: Textbook page references are provided as a guide for answering these questions. A complete answer key is provided to your instructor.

MATCHING

Match the drug name on the right to the drug class on the left.

Drug Class		Drug Name
1. _____ aminoglycosides	a.	piperacillin and tazobactam (Zosyn)
2. _____ carbapenems	b.	co-trimoxazole (Bactrim)
3. _____ cephalosporins	c.	gentamicin
4. _____ macrolides	d.	azithromycin (Zithromax)
5. _____ penicillins	e.	ertapenem (Invanz)
6. _____ quinolones	f.	levofloxacin (Levaquin)
7. _____ sulfonamides	g.	cefepime (Maxipime)

REVIEW QUESTIONS

Scenario: An 89-year-old male patient was admitted to the hospital with urosepsis. He has a history of diabetes, hypertension, hypothyroidism, depression, functional decline, and gastroesophageal reflux disease (GERD).

Explain the major actions and effects of classes of drugs used to treat infectious diseases.

8. Antibiotics from the drug class macrolides have which action on bacteria? *(699)*
   1. They inhibit the ability of the bacteria to synthesize protein.
   2. They weaken the cell wall of the bacteria so that the contents spill out.
   3. They prevent the bacteria from making folic acid.
   4. They inhibit the ability of the bacteria to create a cell wall.
9. Which conditions would aminoglycosides be used to treat? *(Select all that apply.)* *(691)*
   1. Gram-negative bacteria causing meningitis
   2. Chronic urinary tract infections
   3. Latent tuberculosis
   4. Wound infections
   5. Life-threatening septicemia
10. The antimicrobial agents from the drug class carbapenems act on bacteria by: *(693)*
    1. preventing bacteria from making folic acid.

2. inhibiting the ability of the bacteria to create a cell wall.
3. weakening the cell wall of the bacteria so that the contents spill out.
4. inhibiting cell wall synthesis.
11. What is the mechanism of action of the class of antibiotics known as streptogramins? *(706)*
    1. They inhibit protein synthesis in bacterial cells.
    2. They inhibit the bacteria's ability to make folic acid.
    3. They interfere with bacterial DNA.
    4. They destroy the bacterial cell wall.
12. Which class of antimicrobials is chemically related to penicillin and acts by inhibiting cell wall synthesis? *(695)*
    1. Quinolones
    2. Macrolides
    3. Cephalosporins
    4. Streptogramins
13. Which statement best describes the mechanism of action of the quinolones? *(704)*
    1. They inhibit protein synthesis in bacterial cells.
    2. They inhibit the bacteria's ability to make folic acid.
    3. They interfere with bacterial DNA.
    4. They destroy the bacterial cell wall.
14. What is the mechanism of action of amphotericin B? *(721)*
    1. Inhibiting biosynthesis of folic acid
    2. Disruption of the cell membrane of fungal cells

3.   Inhibiting DNA synthesis of the cells
4.   Interfering with the enzyme needed for cell wall generation

15.   Which class of antimicrobials is reserved for serious life-threatening infections that are vancomycin-resistant, and act by inhibiting protein synthesis in bacterial cells? *(706)*
1.   Carbapenems
2.   Streptogramins
3.   Quinolones
4.   Cephalosporins

16.   Which antibiotic is effective against aerobic and anaerobic bacteria, and acts by inhibiting bacterial cell wall synthesis? *(693)*
1.   Levofloxacin
2.   Sulfadiazine
3.   Ertapenem
4.   Gentamicin

List the signs and symptoms of a secondary infection.

17.   The nurse will monitor the patient in the scenario carefully for signs and symptoms of a secondary infection, which will include: *(Select all that apply.)* *(689)*
1.   phlebitis at the IV site.
2.   anal lesions.
3.   severe diarrhea.
4.   tinnitus and progressive hearing loss.
5.   white patches in the oral cavity.

18.   Which measures may be taken by the nurse to minimize the effects of a secondary infection? *(Select all that apply.)* *(689)*
1.   Administer additional antimicrobials effective against the new organism.
2.   Monitor for the development of symptoms of secondary infection.
3.   Obtain cultures as ordered.
4.   Notify the healthcare provider if signs and symptoms of a secondary infection occur.
5.   Hold the prescribed antimicrobial medication when effects are noticed.

19.   After completing education on antibiotic therapy for the patient in the scenario, the nurse knows that more teaching is needed when the patient states: *(698)*
1.   "I should try to avoid people who have an infection like pneumonia."
2.   "I know that my kidneys may be affected with this antibiotic, so I will report any decline in my urine output."
3.   "If I notice any symptoms like sore throat, bruising, or worsening fatigue, I need to report them immediately."
4.   "If I develop any diarrhea, I will just take some over-the-counter Lomotil."

20.   Which symptoms of hepatotoxicity will the patient be able to monitor for after discharge from the hospital? *(Select all that apply.)* *(690)*

1.   Elevated bilirubin
2.   Nausea and vomiting
3.   Jaundice
4.   Hepatomegaly
5.   Anorexia

21.   A patient newly prescribed the cephalosporin Ceclor asked the nurse how she would know if she was experiencing an allergic reaction. The nurse correctly responds: *(689)*
1.   "Most of the time it will just be a rash on your arm."
2.   "The drug Ceclor does not have any allergies associated with it."
3.   "Nausea, vomiting, and diarrhea are the most common symptoms of an allergic reaction."
4.   "Trouble breathing, skin rashes, or facial edema may be symptoms of an allergic reaction."

Describe the signs and symptoms of the common adverse effects of antimicrobial therapy.

22.   Which are common adverse effects often seen with antimicrobial therapy? *(Select all that apply.)* *(689)*
1.   Nausea and vomiting
2.   Secondary infections
3.   Allergies
4.   Constipation
5.   Bleeding tendencies

23.   The patient in the scenario was started on cefepime (Maxipime) for his infection. Which medication prescribed for another clinical condition did the nurse notice was contraindicated with cefepime, requiring notifying the prescriber? *(697)*
1.   Metformin (Glucophage)
2.   Atenolol (Tenormin)
3.   Famotidine (Pepcid)
4.   Levothyroxine

24.   The severe adverse reaction of nephrotoxicity from antimicrobial therapy can be monitored by which laboratory results? *(Select all that apply.)* *(689)*
1.   AST
2.   Creatinine
3.   WBC
4.   BUN
5.   Hgb

Describe the nursing assessments and interventions for the common adverse effects associated with antimicrobial agents: allergic reaction, nephrotoxicity, ototoxicity, and hepatotoxicity.

25.   A patient who was being treated for cellulitis returned to the clinic with complaints of his arm looking sunburnt and developing patches that itch after being outside. The nurse recognizes these symptoms as: *(690)*
1.   blood dyscrasia.
2.   photosensitivity.
3.   nephrotoxicity.
4.   secondary infection.

26. Prior to administration of a carbapenem, what premedication assessments should be performed? *(Select all that apply.) (693)*
    1. Check hydration status.
    2. Check vital signs.
    3. Assess basic mental status.
    4. Check any allergies specifically to penicillin and cephalosporins.
    5. Determine that the organism being treated is *Candida albicans.*

27. The nurse was performing a premedication assessment before therapy with cephalosporins on a patient. Which condition observed in the patient would indicate the drug should be held and the healthcare provider notified? *(695)*
    1. Low urine output and concentrated urine
    2. Onychomycosis of the toenail
    3. Oral candidiasis
    4. Exophthalmos

28. Which antimicrobial agent would be contraindicated in a patient who will be receiving neuromuscular blockade for a surgical procedure? *(693)*
    1. Sulfonamides (i.e., sulfadiazine)
    2. Quinolones (i.e., norfloxacin)
    3. Aminoglycosides (neomycin)
    4. Carbapenems (ertapenem)

29. Why is it essential to report the occurrence of severe diarrhea with antibiotic therapy? *(694)*
    1. This may mean that the drug is not being absorbed any further.
    2. This may indicate drug-induced pseudomembranous colitis.
    3. This would indicate that an allergic response has occurred.
    4. This would indicate nephrotoxicity.

30. The assessment data that the nurse will monitor for the patient in the scenario, who has now been receiving antibiotics for his infection, include noting: *(Select all that apply.) (688)*
    1. any photosensitivity.
    2. changes in laboratory results (i.e., WBC).
    3. any allergic reactions.
    4. when his last vaccination for flu was given.
    5. any symptoms that may indicate a secondary infection is developing.

31. When administering aminoglycosides to a patient, what does the nurse assess? *(Select all that apply.) (692)*
    1. Whether anesthesia was administered to the patient within the past 48–72 hours
    2. Any development of dizziness, tinnitus, and progressive hearing loss
    3. Any allergy to penicillin, because patients allergic to penicillin are allergic to aminoglycosides
    4. Any history of renal disease
    5. Adequate hydration status related to any nausea and vomiting

Cite the primary uses for antibiotic agents, antitubercular agents, antifungal agents, and antiviral agents.

32. Antimicrobial agents can be classified according to the type of pathogenic organism such as: *(Select all that apply.) (687)*
    1. pollen.
    2. fungus.
    3. cerumen.
    4. viruses.
    5. bacteria.

33. The therapeutic outcome expected from tigecycline (Tygacil) is elimination of bacterial infection, which is related to what fact? *(697)*
    1. It is approved for use in children and adolescents.
    2. It is effective against viruses.
    3. It is a bacteriostatic antibiotic.
    4. It is susceptible to the mechanisms that cause resistance to the tetracyclines.

34. Which infections can macrolides be used for? *(Select all that apply.) (699)*
    1. Prophylactic before surgery
    2. Respiratory
    3. Sexually transmitted infection
    4. Gastrointestinal tract
    5. Skin and soft-tissue infections

35. Which are clinical uses of penicillins? *(Select all that apply.) (702)*
    1. Treatment of middle-ear infection
    2. Treatment of urinary tract infections
    3. Prophylactic antibiotic for syphilis and gonorrhea
    4. Treatment of pneumonia
    5. Prophylactic antibiotic for meningitis

36. Because the sulfonamides inhibit bacterial biosynthesis of folic acid, which needs to be monitored periodically when patients are on these antibiotics? *(707)*
    1. PT and platelets
    2. Creatinine and BUN
    3. RBC and WBC (with differential) counts
    4. Electrolytes

37. What are the effects of administering tetracyclines during pregnancy? *(709)*
    1. They may cause dental caries.
    2. They may cause enamel staining.
    3. They may cause birth defects.
    4. They may cause preterm labor.

38. The nurse preparing isoniazid and rifampin to be administered to a patient knows that these antibiotics are being given for the treatment of: *(710-711)*
    1. syphilis.
    2. trichinosis.
    3. tuberculosis.
    4. cellulitis.

39. What is ketoconazole used to treat? *(Select all that apply.)* **(746)**
    1. Chromomycosis
    2. Candidiasis
    3. Onychomycosis
    4. Histoplasmosis
    5. Coccidioidomycosis

Nutrition

Answer Key: Textbook page references are provided as a guide for answering these questions. A complete answer key is provided to your instructor.

MATCHING
Match the definition on the right with the key term on the left.

Key Term		Definition
1. _____	Dietary Reference Intakes (DRIs)	a. the highest level of daily nutrient intake that is likely to pose no risk of adverse health effects
2. _____	Estimated Average Requirement (EAR)	b. a list of average daily dietary intake level that meets the nutrient requirements of almost all healthy individuals in a group
3. _____	Recommended Dietary Allowances (RDAs)	c. the most common form of malnutrition in hospitalized patients
4. _____	Adequate Intake (AI)	d. the average dietary energy intake that is predicted to maintain energy balance in healthy adults
5. _____	Tolerable Upper Intake Level (UL)	e. provides quantitative estimates of nutrient intakes for planning and assessing diets
6. _____	Estimated Energy Requirement (EER)	f. a protein deficiency that develops when little or no protein is in the diet
7. _____	marasmus	g. a nutrient intake value that is estimated to meet the requirement of half of the healthy individuals in a group
8. _____	kwashiorkor	h. a value based on observed or experimentally determined approximations of nutrient intake by a group of healthy people

REVIEW QUESTIONS

Scenario: A 75-year-old female patient came to the clinic with complaints of fatigue and increasing weakness. She has been losing weight, has poor appetite, and noticed that her hair is dry and falls out easily.

Identify sources of dietary fiber and dietary fats.

9. What are the essential macronutrients needed by the body? *(Select all that apply.)* **(735)**
   1. Fiber
   2. Carbohydrates
   3. Water
   4. Proteins
   5. Fats

10. The nurse educating a patient on his diet with regards to the recommended primary sources of fats, suggested which foods are healthy? *(Select all that apply.)* **(738)**
    1. Coconut oil
    2. Olive oil
    3. Low-fat milk
    4. Avocados
    5. Soybean oil

11. Which fat source is of concern because it has no known nutritional benefit? **(736)**
    1. Saturated fats
    2. Polyunsaturated fats
    3. Trans fats
    4. Monounsaturated fats

12. Which foods are considered good fiber sources? *(Select all that apply.)* **(737-738)**
    1. Ice cream
    2. Legumes
    3. Rice
    4. Sweet potatoes
    5. Cereal bran

Differentiate between fat-soluble and water-soluble vitamins and discuss their functions.

13. Which vitamins are water-soluble? *(Select all that apply.)* **(743)**
    1. Niacin
    2. Ascorbic acid

3. Cyanocobalamin
4. Retinol
5. Phytonadione

14. The nurse was administering cholecalciferol to a patient who asks what it is. The nurse responds by stating: *(735)*
    1. "It is one of those water-soluble vitamins that are necessary in your diet."
    2. "I believe this is vitamin E."
    3. "This is vitamin D, which helps regulate calcium and phosphorus metabolism."
    4. "This is another name for vitamin B."

15. The nurse discussing with a patient which foods contain vitamin B_2 will provide further teaching after the patient states: *(743)*
    1. "I can get vitamin B_2 in my diet by eating pork, peas, and dry beans."
    2. "If I eat green leafy vegetables, fruit, and eggs I will being getting some vitamin B_2."
    3. "I know that vitamin B_2 is important because it is needed for normal cell function."
    4. "Another name for vitamin B_2 is riboflavin."

Discuss the functions of minerals in the body.

16. Which mineral found in drinking water and seafood is essential for bone and tooth structure? *(744)*
    1. Chromium
    2. Chlorine
    3. Fluorine
    4. Iodine

17. Which mineral found in grains, green leafy vegetables, nuts, and legumes is essential for protein synthesis and nerve transmission? *(744)*
    1. Magnesium
    2. Manganese
    3. Phosphorus
    4. Chromium

18. Which mineral found in whole grains, cereals, green vegetables, and tea is essential for fat and connective tissue synthesis? *(744)*
    1. Calcium
    2. Manganese
    3. Magnesium
    4. Cobalt

Describe physical changes associated with a malnourished state.

19. The nurse found the following assessment characteristics in the patient in the scenario and noted which ones that indicate a malnourished state? *(Select all that apply.)* *(746)*
    1. Weight loss
    2. Elevated temperature
    3. Dry hair that easily falls out
    4. Crackles in lung fields
    5. Fatigue and weakness

20. What laboratory studies can be used to assess lean body mass? *(Select all that apply.)* *(745)*

1. Retinol-binding protein
2. Albumin
3. Prealbumin
4. Transferrin
5. Ferritin

21. When providing patient teaching about kwashiorkor, which statements does the nurse include? *(Select all that apply.)* *(745)*
    1. "It occurs because of a fat deficiency in the diet."
    2. "Patients with this condition are often difficult to recognize because they appear to be well-nourished."
    3. "Patients with this condition receive adequate carbohydrates in the diet."
    4. "Patients with this condition receive adequate protein in the diet."
    5. "Patients are usually dehydrated when they have this condition."

Discuss nursing assessments and interventions required during the administration of enteral nutrition.

22. What are the general routines nurses use to monitor tube feedings? *(Select all that apply.)* *(747)*
    1. Changing the tube feeding bag every 4 hours
    2. Checking tube placement
    3. Monitoring for diarrhea or cramping
    4. Checking residual volumes of enteral feedings
    5. Keeping formulas at room temperature when not in use

23. What assessments does the nurse perform prior to administering enteral nutrition? *(Select all that apply.)* *(747)*
    1. Assess for lactose intolerance.
    2. Assess bowel function.
    3. Assess daily weights.
    4. Assess the patency of the IV.
    5. Check laboratory results of Hgb, ALT, AST, and albumin.

24. How does the nurse administer a tube feeding that is ordered to be given intermittently? *(750)*
    1. Administer 200 mL over 30 minutes using gravity.
    2. Slowly administer over 12 to 24 hours using a pump.
    3. Administer 200 mL over 5 minutes using a syringe.
    4. Administer 200 mL over 10 minutes using a pump.

Describe the advantages and disadvantages of nutrition by PPN and CPN.

25. What is the difference between PPN solutions and CPN solutions? *(Select all that apply.)* *(752)*
    1. CPN is used for patients who need nutritional support for 3 to 4 weeks; PPN is used for patients who require long-term nutritional support.

2. PPN solutions consist of 5–10% dextrose; CPN consists of 15–25% glucose.
3. CPN solutions must be administered through a central venous access line; PPN solutions may be administered through a peripheral line.
4. CPN solutions need to be run by an infusion pump; PPN solutions can be either gravity or infusion pump.
5. PPN solutions consist of 2–5% amino acids; CPN solutions consist of 3.5–15% amino acids.

26. Which adverse effects of parenteral feedings should be reported to the healthcare provider? *(Select all that apply.) (753)*
    1. Respiratory difficulty
    2. Rash, chills, and fever
    3. Hypoglycemia and/or hyperglycemia
    4. Infusion pump alarm for air in line
    5. 50 mL of solution remains in the bag after 24 hours

27. The nurse was discussing the advantages of enteral nutrition over parenteral nutrition with a patient who was going home with a gastrostomy port. Additional instruction was required after the patient stated: *(749)*
    1. "I know that this feeding will help stimulate my GI tract."
    2. "As I understand it, there is less of a chance of infection with this tube."
    3. "I understand these feedings are more expensive than if I had an IV drip for nutrition."
    4. "I will be getting all my nutrition through these feedings."

Herbal and Dietary Supplement Therapy

Answer Key: Textbook page references are provided as a guide for answering these questions. A complete answer key is provided to your instructor.

MATCHING

Match the supplement on the right with its use on the left.

	Use		Supplement
1.	_____ a common beverage used to improve cognitive performance and stimulate the CNS	a.	aloe
2.	_____ research supports that it reduces cholesterol and triglyceride levels	b.	chamomile
		c.	ephedra
3.	_____ used as a digestive aid for bloating, and an antispasmodic and antiinflammatory of the GI tract	d.	feverfew
4.	_____ used to alleviate nausea and vomiting from a variety of causes	e.	garlic
		f.	ginger
5.	_____ used primarily as an adjunctive therapy for chronic heart failure	g.	ginkgo
6.	_____ used to increase the body's resistance to stress	h.	ginseng
		i.	green tea
7.	_____ frequently used as a coingredient in skin care products for healing sunburn	j.	St. John's wort
8.	_____ used for restlessness and it may promote sleep	k.	valerian
		l.	CoQ10
9.	_____ used to reduce the frequency and severity of migraine headaches		
10.	_____ used to treat short-term memory loss, headaches, dizziness, tinnitus, and emotional instability		
11.	_____ used orally to treat mild depression and to heal wounds		
12.	_____ used as a bronchodilator for asthma; a nasal decongestant; and a CNS stimulant		

REVIEW QUESTIONS

Scenario: A 52-year-old woman came to the clinic complaining of joint pain, especially in her knees. She was told she may be getting degenerative joint disease. She told the nurse that she has been taking ginger and black cohosh.

Summarize the primary actions and potential uses of the herbal and dietary supplement products cited.

13. When a patient is taking aloe, it is most important for the nurse to assess the patient for the development of which condition? *(758)*
    1. Infection
    2. Hypertension
    3. Hypokalemia
    4. Hypoglycemia

14. The nurse tells the patient in the scenario when the use of black cohosh would be contraindicated by stating: *(758)*
    1. "Black cohosh should not be used by patients who have arthritis conditions."
    2. "Black cohosh should not be used in the first two trimesters of pregnancy."
    3. "Black cohosh should not be used by patients who are immunocompromised."
    4. "Black cohosh should not be used by patients who are allergic to ragweed or asters."

15. What are common uses for chamomile? *(Select all that apply.)* *(759)*
    1. Alleviate nausea and vomiting
    2. Digestive agent for bloating
    3. An antiinflammatory for skin irritation
    4. An antispasmodic for menstrual cramps

5. A mouthwash for minor mouth irritation or gum infections

16. A patient with which condition is most likely to benefit from the administration of echinacea? *(759)*
    1. Acquired immunodeficiency syndrome (AIDS)
    2. Multiple sclerosis
    3. Viral respiratory tract infection
    4. Systemic lupus erythematosus

17. Which herb is most commonly used in the treatment of asthma? *(760)*
    1. Ephedra
    2. Echinacea
    3. Chamomile
    4. Goldenseal

18. What are common uses for feverfew? *(Select all that apply.) (761)*
    1. Reduce the frequency and severity of migraine headaches
    2. Improve digestion and gastroesophageal reflux disease (GERD) symptoms
    3. Alleviate nausea and vomiting
    4. Treatment of rheumatoid arthritis
    5. Reduce allergic response to ragweed

19. What common use for garlic is supported by scientific literature? *(761)*
    1. Improve digestion and GERD symptoms
    2. Reduce cholesterol and triglycerides
    3. Alleviate nausea and vomiting
    4. Reduce fever and inflammation

20. The patient in the scenario was asking the nurse what effects ginger has as an herbal preparation. Which statement would be an appropriate response from the nurse? *(Select all that apply.) (762)*
    1. "Ginger has no medicinal effects, so it basically works like a placebo."
    2. "Ginger has been used for centuries to alleviate nausea and vomiting."
    3. "Ginger has some modest effects in reducing the inflammation associated with rheumatoid arthritis."
    4. "Ginger works as an aphrodisiac."
    5. "Ginger has been known to reduce allergic reactions in patients with hayfever."

21. What is *Ginkgo biloba* extract commonly used for? *(Select all that apply.) (762)*
    1. To improve hearing in patients with hearing impairment due to poor circulation to the ears.
    2. To increase cerebral blood flow, particularly in geriatric patients.
    3. To improve erectile dysfunction secondary to antidepressant therapy.
    4. To improve walking distance in patients with intermittent claudication.
    5. To improve eyesight in patients with vision impairment due to poor circulation to the eyes.

22. Which herb is also known by other names that include *red berry, tartar root, five fingers,* and *aralia cinquefoil*? *(763)*

1. Goldenseal
2. Ginseng
3. Valerian
4. Feverfew

23. Which herb has its active ingredients contained in plant alkaloids? *(764)*
    1. St. John's wort
    2. Ginseng
    3. Goldenseal
    4. Green tea

24. Of the following ingredients that are active in green tea, which causes the adverse effects such as anxiety, nervousness, and insomnia? *(764)*
    1. Caffeine
    2. Gallic acid
    3. Catechins
    4. Ascorbic acid

25. Which herb is used for treatment of mild depression? *(765)*
    1. Valerian
    2. Green tea
    3. St. John's wort
    4. Ginseng

26. Which statements does the nurse include when teaching a patient about St. John's wort? *(Select all that apply.) (765)*
    1. "The active ingredients of St. John's wort are unknown."
    2. "St. John's wort may cause photosensitivity, so individuals using it should avoid overexposure to the sun."
    3. "Patients who take other serotonin stimulants should not take St. John's wort without consulting their healthcare provider."
    4. "St. John's wort is a safe drug for anyone with depression."
    5. "There are no adverse effects associated with the use of St. John's wort."

27. Which are common uses for valerian? *(Select all that apply.) (765)*
    1. Laxative
    2. Reduce inflammation
    3. Restlessness
    4. Sleep aid
    5. Digestive aid

28. The provitamin coenzyme Q_{10} can be found in every living cell and accumulates in high levels in organs that have high energy requirements such as the: *(Select all that apply.) (766)*
    1. liver.
    2. brain.
    3. pancreas.
    4. lung.
    5. heart.

29. Which herbal preparation is thought to enhance muscle performance for short bouts of intense exercise? *(766)*

1. Gamma-hydroxybutyrate
2. Coenzyme Q$_{10}$
3. Melatonin
4. Creatine

30. Why is gamma-hydroxybutyrate (GHB) available as a prescription-only product used for narcolepsy? *(767)*
    1. The adverse effects are hypertension and tachycardia.
    2. The effects of its blood-thinning properties make it too dangerous.
    3. It easily produces symptoms of nausea, vomiting, and diarrhea.
    4. It has been used as a "date rape" drug added to alcoholic drinks.

31. Which herbal compound is found in tomatoes, watermelon, and pink grapefruit? *(768)*
    1. Lycopene
    2. Melatonin
    3. Ginseng
    4. Chamomile

32. Which preparation is naturally produced from serotonin and secreted by the pineal gland? *(768)*
    1. Omega-3 fatty acids
    2. Policosanol
    3. Melatonin
    4. Lycopene

33. Which action is policosanol used to produce? *(769)*
    1. Lower cholesterol levels
    2. Lower blood pressure
    3. Decrease pulse rate
    4. Lower blood sugar

34. Which are sources of omega-3 fatty acids? *(Select all that apply.)* *(769)*
    1. Sardines
    2. Soybeans
    3. Flaxseed
    4. Peanuts
    5. Tuna

35. Which conditions are possible indications for the use of S-adenosylmethionine (SAM-e)? *(Select all that apply.)* *(770)*
    1. Depression
    2. Osteoarthritis

3. Diabetes mellitus
4. Fibromyalgia
5. Infection

Describe the interactions between commonly used herbal and dietary supplement products and prescription medications.

36. The patient in the scenario is on hormone replacement therapy to treat symptoms associated with menopause and to prevent osteoporosis. She also takes medication to control high blood pressure. She asks the nurse about the risks of taking black cohosh. What is the best response by the nurse? *(759)*
    1. "Studies have found that black cohosh is an excellent herb for women to treat symptoms of menopause that are not controlled by hormone replacement therapy."
    2. "High blood pressure will be lowered with the use of black cohosh, so you won't need to take your high blood pressure pills any longer."
    3. "Black cohosh works by stimulating the body to produce its own natural testosterone."
    4. "Black cohosh may cause added antihypertensive effects when taken with medication to lower blood pressure. Consult your healthcare provider before adding black cohosh to your treatment regimen."

37. Which herbal supplement affects platelet aggregation and therefore should be used with caution for patients taking antiplatelet medications? *(762)*
    1. Ephedra
    2. Garlic
    3. Melatonin
    4. Black cohosh

38. The nurse needs to caution patients who drink alcohol or take benzodiazepines and sleep aids that the adverse effect of CNS depression may occur with the addition of: *(768)*
    1. policosanol.
    2. creatine.
    3. melatonin.
    4. omega-3 fatty acids.

Substance Abuse

Answer Key: Textbook page references are provided as a guide for answering these questions. A complete answer key is provided to your instructor.

MATCHING
Match the slang drug name on the right with the substances of abuse on the left.

Substance of Abuse		Slang Name
1. _____ heroin	a.	acid
2. _____ nicotine	b.	blast
3. _____ cocaine	c.	booze
4. _____ marijuana	d.	weed
5. _____ LSD	e.	angel dust
6. _____ PCP	f.	China white
7. _____ alcohol	g.	chew

REVIEW QUESTIONS

Scenario: A 26-year-old woman came into the clinic for a prenatal exam and was obviously intoxicated.

Identify the differences between mild, moderate, and severe substance abuse disorder.

8. The term *social impairment* is described as having which components? *(Select all that apply.)* **(773)**
   1. Development of withdrawal symptoms when blood levels decline
   2. Continuation of substance use in spite of persistent social problems
   3. Craving exhibited by a powerful urge for the substance
   4. Reduction or cessation of important social, occupational, or recreational pursuits because of substance use
   5. Failure to fulfill major role responsibilities at work, school, or home due to recurrent substance use

9. When four or five symptoms of substance use disorders are present, the patient is classified as having: **(772)**
   1. mild substance abuse disorder.
   2. moderate substance abuse disorder.
   3. severe substance abuse disorder.
   4. a true addictive substance disorder.

10. What symptoms are included in the description of a severe substance abuse disorder? *(Select all that apply.)* **(772)**
    1. An overwhelming compulsion to use the substance
    2. Feeling depressed when not using the substance
    3. A tolerance for higher amounts of the substance
    4. The use of illicit substances
    5. Withdrawal symptoms on discontinuation of the substance

Differentiate between the screening instruments for substance use disorders.

11. What questionnaire will the nurse use as a quick screening instrument for assessment of alcohol abuse for the patient in the scenario? **(776)**
    1. MMPI
    2. API
    3. CAGE
    4. DUSI

12. What is one disadvantage of many of the screening instruments used for assessment of substance abuse? **(778)**
    1. They were developed using adult male patients and have not been validated in other populations.
    2. They have many lengthy questions and are not specific enough to detect the difference between excessive drinking and alcoholism.
    3. They have been designed as self-assessment tools and require the use of a computer.
    4. They cannot differentiate between alcohol problems or drug problems.

13. Screening instruments used by healthcare professionals for patients who are suspected of substance abuse are divided into which four categories? *(Select all that apply.)* **(776)**
    1. Lengthy drug abuse screening
    2. Alcohol abuse screening
    3. Comprehensive drug abuse screening
    4. Brief drug abuse screening
    5. Drug and alcohol abuse screening for use with adolescents

Cite the responsibilities of professionals who suspect substance abuse by a colleague.

14. What is the prevalence of substance abuse by healthcare professionals? *(778)*
    1. Much lower than the general population
    2. Much higher than the general population
    3. Similar to the general population
    4. Unheard of in this profession

15. What should a healthcare professional do if he or she suspects a colleague of being impaired on the job? *(778)*
    1. Do nothing, but keep an eye on the colleague.
    2. Confront the individual about the suspicion.
    3. Make a confidential report to the supervisor.
    4. Inform all coworkers about the situation.

16. A nurse was discussing her suspicions about a coworker to her supervisor and asked if the coworker was going to lose her job. What is the best response by the supervisor? *(778)*
    1. "Yes, unfortunately that is the way it works. We cannot have someone impaired on the job."
    2. "No, not at this point. The next step is to have this person enter a treatment program."
    3. "No, we cannot afford to fire anyone at this time; we are too understaffed."
    4. "Yes, but she could always reapply for the job after she has been out for a year."

Explain the primary long-term goals in the treatment of substance abuse.

17. When providing teaching to the patient in the scenario about the effects of substance use and abuse with pregnancy, which statements does the nurse include? *(Select all that apply.)* *(787)*
    1. "Using alcohol and drugs while pregnant has a strong likelihood of harming the baby after birth."
    2. "Infants of drug addicts must be monitored closely for symptoms of withdrawal after delivery."
    3. "Using alcohol and drugs during pregnancy has a high likelihood of causing the need for induction of pregnancy due to the fetus being postterm."
    4. "Alcohol and drug use during pregnancy has been associated with potentially fatal bleeding disorders."
    5. "Babies of mothers who used alcohol during pregnancy have a higher incidence of behavioral problems later in life."

18. What are the long-term goals in treating substance abuse? *(Select all that apply.)* *(779)*
    1. Maintenance of social functioning
    2. Reduction in the severity of relapse
    3. Reduction in the frequency of relapse
    4. Abstinence in the use of the substance being abused
    5. Reduction in the use of the substance being abused

19. When patients are participating in organizations such as Alcoholics Anonymous or Narcotics Anonymous, what types of resources are available to them? *(Select all that apply.)* *(779)*
    1. Advice on abstinence
    2. Money for expenses
    3. Role modeling
    4. 24-hour help available when a craving occurs
    5. Networking

Identify the withdrawal symptoms for major substances that are commonly abused.

20. Which are signs and symptoms of opioid intoxication? *(Select all that apply.)* *(782)*
    1. Apathy
    2. Inappropriate behaviors
    3. Miosis, slurred speech
    4. Avoidance of dangerous situations
    5. Impaired judgment

21. What drug class is used to treat alcohol withdrawal symptoms? *(780)*
    1. Adrenergic agents
    2. Benzodiazepines
    3. Cholinergic agents
    4. Anticholinergic agents

22. When working with a patient who is withdrawing from long-term use of amphetamines, the nurse expects the patient to exhibit which signs/symptoms? *(Select all that apply.)* *(784)*
    1. Severe depression
    2. Fatigue
    3. Loss of memory
    4. Inability to manipulate information
    5. Insomnia

Miscellaneous Agents

Answer Key: Textbook page references are provided as a guide for answering these questions. A complete answer key is provided to your instructor.

MATCHING

Match the correct drug use on the right with the drug name on the left. Drug uses on the right can be used more than once.

Drug Name

1. _____ allopurinol
2. _____ colchicine
3. _____ donepezil
4. _____ memantine
5. _____ probenecid

Drug Use

a. used to prevent or relieve attacks of gout
b. used to treat hyperuricemia
c. used in patients with Alzheimer's–associated dementia to improve cognitive skills

REVIEW QUESTIONS

Scenario: A 54-year-old male patient comes into the clinic complaining of pain in the great toe on the left foot. He was diagnosed with gout and prescribed colchicine.

Summarize the primary actions and potential uses of the miscellaneous agents cited.

6. What is the primary therapeutic outcome of colchicine therapy? *(794)*
   1. Dissolve uric acid crystals
   2. Inhibit the production of uric acid
   3. Decrease the amount of uric acid in the blood or urine
   4. Eliminate joint pain secondary to acute gout attack
7. What is the primary action of donepezil (Aricept)? *(795)*
   1. It inhibits acetylcholinesterase, the enzyme that breaks down acetylcholine.
   2. It allows norepinephrine to accumulate at the neuron synapses.
   3. It prevents the loss of cholinergic neurons.
   4. It activates acetylcholinesterase, the enzyme that breaks down acetylcholine.
8. What is the primary therapeutic outcome of memantine (Namenda)? *(796)*
   1. The prevention or slowing of the neurodegeneration of Alzheimer's disease
   2. The improvement of cognitive skills

3. The enhancement of muscle tone
4. The improvement of mobility and coordination

9. How does probenecid prevent acute attacks of gouty arthritis? *(796)*
   1. It dissolves uric acid crystals.
   2. It inhibits the production of uric acid.
   3. It enhances the excretion of uric acid by the kidneys.
   4. It relieves the pain in joints affected by gout.

Describe patient education needed when miscellaneous agents are used.

10. After completing the education for the patient in the scenario on the use of colchicine, the nurse will need to provide further education when the patient states: *(794)*
    1. "I need to take this to prevent an attack of gout."
    2. "My joint swelling will subside within 12 hours."
    3. "It will take from 48 to 72 hours before I will get any pain relief."
    4. "I know I can take a dose every 3 days to prevent an attack of gout."
11. The nurse has provided patient teaching for probenecid therapy. Which statement by the patient indicates that more teaching is needed? *(796)*
    1. "This drug works on the tissues of my great toe, where I usually get the gout, to get rid of the problem."

2. "I can expect that the incidence of gout attacks may increase for the first few months of therapy with this drug."

3. "I will tell my healthcare provider if I develop vomiting that looks like coffee grounds."

4. "If I develop a rash, I will tell my healthcare provider because this most likely means that I have an allergy to this drug."

12. Which statements does the nurse include when teaching a patient and family about donepezil (Aricept)? *(Select all that apply.)* **(795)**

1. "Notify your healthcare provider if your pulse is fewer than 60 beats per minute."

2. "Discontinue the drug if you develop diarrhea early in the treatment program."

3. "This drug will prevent your disease from getting worse."

4. "You may feel a little nauseated when first taking this medication, but this usually subsides after 2 to 3 weeks of therapy."

5. "Donepezil must be taken on an empty stomach."